OSCEs for Students, Second E

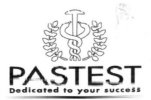

PASTEST
Dedicated to your success

OSCEs for Medical Students, Volume 2
Second Edition

Adam Feather
John S P Lumley
Ramanathan Visvanathan

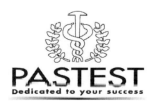

PASTEST
Dedicated to your success

© 2004 PASTEST Ltd
Egerton Court
Parkgate Estate
Knutsford
Cheshire
WA16 8DX

Telephone: 01565 752000

First published 2004

ISBN: 1 904627 10 2

A catalogue record for this book is available from the British Library.

The information contained within this book was obtained by the authors from reliable sources. However, while every effort has been made to ensure its accuracy, no responsibility for loss, damage or injury occasioned to any person acting or refraining from action as a result of information contained herein can be accepted by the publishers or authors.

PasTest Revision Books and Intensive Courses
PasTest has been established in the field of postgraduate medical education since 1972, providing revision books and intensive study courses for doctors preparing for their professional examinations.

Books and courses are available for the following specialties:
MRCGP, MRCP Parts 1 and 2, MRCPCH Parts 1 and 2, MRCPsych, MRCS, MRCOG Parts 1 and 2, DRCOG, FRCA, PLAB Parts 1 and 2.

For further details contact:
PasTest, Knutsford, Cheshire WA16 7BR
Tel: 01565 752000   Fax: 01565 650264
www.pastest.co.uk   enquiries@pastest.co.uk

Text prepared by Carnegie Book Production, Lancaster
Printed and bound in Europe by The Alden Group

Contents

OSCE Stations

Answers with Explanations and Comments

Contributors

Adam Feather MB MRCP
Senior Lecturer in Medical Education
St Bartholomew's and The Royal London Hospital Medical School
Consultant Physician
Newham Healthcare Trust
London

John S P Lumley MS FRCS
Professor of Vascular Surgery
University of London
Honorary Consultant Surgeon
Great Ormond Street Children's Hospital
Medical College and Hospital of St Bartholomew, London
Member of Council, Royal College of Surgeons of England
Past World President, International College of Surgeons

Ramanathan Visvanathan BM BCh FRCS ILTM
Consultant Surgeon
Bronglais General Hospital
Aberystwyth
SY23 1ER
And Breast Test Wales, Swansea
Honorary Lecturer, University of Wales College of Medicine
Surgical Tutor, Royal College of Surgeons of England

Angela Hall BSc Postgrad DipSoc
Senior Lecturer in Clinical Communications
Department of Medical Health Care Education
St George's Hospital Medical School
Cranmer Terrace
Tooting
London
SW17 0RE

Acknowledgements

These volumes would not have reached their present high standards without the excellent contribution made by Angela Hall, Senior Lecturer in Communication Skills at St George's Hospital Medical School. Her expert advice on the process elements of all the communication skills stations have improved the quality and have helped to produce stations which truly reflect those used at the majority of UK medical schools at final MBBS. Whilst the style of OSCE checklists will no doubt evolve over the next few years the elements she has included will not. We are very grateful to her for her expert contribution.

Preface

Followers of recent literature on the assessment of undergraduate medical training could be excused for thinking that traditional methods were incomplete, if not arbitrary, and that potentially harmful doctors were being let loose on an unsuspecting public. This opinion is based on the immeasurable nature of 'gut feeling' in the marking of an essay and assessing clinical competence. The application of objective measurement in qualifying examinations does add credibility to their outcome.

Every examination must be fair and favour the well-prepared, ie valid and reliable. We have discussed the relative merits of essays, SAQs and MCQs elsewhere, this book, (and its companion volumes), is directed at the use of OSCEs in medicine. It provides a means of assessing practical procedures and communication skills, as well as knowledge and attitudes in most aspects of training.

The book is aimed at students preparing for their exit examination and will provide experience in this now widely-used examination technique. The book will also help those setting OSCE questions, providing a template onto which they can develop their own themes. OSCEs can assess history, examination, investigation and treatment of disease, together with practical techniques. OSCE stations can also obtain information on attitudes, interpersonal skills and ethical opinions. Some of these stations require the use of standard patients, manikin and videos. Although these media are not all reproduceable in a text book, advice is given on the way to deal with the likely questions, techniques and style of stations that may be encountered. It indicates what the examiner is looking for and how marks are being allocated for the approach to a patient and empathy with their problem. A correct diagnosis is not necessarily the key to obtaining a satisfactory mark: always remember to read the instructions very carefully.

The book follows a systems approach and each chapter includes questions from each type of OSCE station. Space is left for the student to respond to each question. Answers and additional advice are given in a separate section, allowing the students to assess their performance and identify areas needing further attention. In keeping with other books in the series, a revision checklist is given, and mock examinations are laid out: these latter can be undertaken within a prescribed time schedule and used for self-assessment.

Preface to Second Edition

A chapter of paediatric stations and an extended chapter in obstetrics and gynaecology have been added in these new editions, increasing the series to three volumes. At the request of students, checklists have been included at the beginning of each chapter and there have been minor stylistic changes.

The marking system in most undergraduate examinations is item-based, although many schools are moving towards the standard postgraduate domain-based assessment, such as of generic skills and examining a region of the body; the text reflects these changing practices.

An interesting and desirable development has been the move back towards structured short cases, with emphasis on diagnostic skills, rather than process. The text also reflects these changes, as seen from the additional examiner's questions in many stations.

Units have not been included in the questions but tables of normal values are included at the beginning of each volume.

Introduction

Traditional methods of assessing knowledge and clinical skills have been based on the essay and MCQ, for written tests, and the long cases, short cases and the viva for practical aspects. These forms of assessment have been extensively challenged as to their ability to test and rank students. The essay has come under the greatest criticism but the long and short cases have also been questioned as to their objectivity and reliability. Marking a viva can be very subjective and it provides a very patchy assessment of the curriculum.

Objective structured clinical examinations (OSCEs) have been designed to provide a broader coverage of knowledge and skills in a quantifiable, valid and reliable form. They aim to assess interpretive skills, as well as factual recall; they include task-orientated items and they can examine a candidate's powers of decision making and their behavioural attitude in simulated professional practice. The overall effect is to provide a more valid assessment of candidates for their subsequent clinical practice.

The OSCE comprises a number of stations, through which a group of students rotate. The number of students in the examination usually matches the number of stations, so that by the end of the examination, each student has visited every station. There may be more stations than candidates without disturbing the organisation of the examination. Usually the time allowed for each station is the same throughout but it can be increased by inserting rest or preparatory stations before a longer question. Rest stations may also be used to provide natural breaks and to increase the number of candidates being examined at any one time.

The time at a station is usually at least three minutes, five minutes being common; 24 stations are available for a two hour examination. For an examination to be statistically reliable there must be a minimum of 17–20 stations. Formative assessments may use a few selected stations (eg 5–10). The design of OSCE questions is usually only limited by the ingenuity of the examiners. However, questions should examine a specific part of the curriculum, rather than just an ability to respond to the style of the examination. Students should be exposed to all proposed designs of question format before the final examination.

Each station of an OSCE should assess a discrete skill. This may be a basic test of practical ability or knowledge, or involve a higher level of thinking. It is wise to have a range of difficulty to help discriminate within a group. A number of questions are included to assess core knowledge: all students are expected to pass these stations. The clinical skills of diagnosis and treatment can be divided up into:

- taking a history
- performing an examination
- requesting appropriate investigations
- making the diagnosis
- assessing the severity of the disease
- prescribing treatment.

The latter should incorporate all aspects of care, including medicine, surgery, nursing and other medical and paramedical disciplines.

The history may be taken from a standardised patient (SP), or presented as a written scenario or a video. SPs may be simulated or actual patients. In the former, a well individual is trained to simulate a patient's illness in a standard way, portraying a patient's problems. Some training is usually required for actual patients, to ensure that the main points are brought out on request and that a history can be covered fully within the time allowed for that station. Simulated patients are usually actors, although sometimes students may act as SPs. In so doing students learn the evaluation process by direct observation and listening to presentations. These stations are usually manned by an examiner who is watching and listening, not only to the style of questioning, but also to student/patient interrelationships, their conversational skills, interpersonal skills, behaviour, attitude and psychomotor assessment. SPs are often asked to give their marks on the student encounter. Written scenarios can form the basis of subsequent questions, along the line of structured answer questions. They can test factual knowledge, understanding and cognitive skills but assess clinical competencies to a variable extent. Well-trained actors can become skilled historians and very persuasive patients, such as when replicating a psychiatric disturbance, although the latter are often more effectively covered with video sequences.

Examination of a patient in a manned station is a very valuable form of assessment. However, it also presents a great problem to the examiner, since very few conditions can be repeatedly examined for two hours at a time, and the number of conditions that can be easily replicated is limited, particularly if there are a number of groups of students being examined simultaneously or consecutively. Fit models can be used for the demonstration of a normal examination and normal anatomy or, alternatively, manikins can be available to assess specific examination techniques such as rectal and vaginal assessment.

A text book has difficulty in reproducing a history and examination, in view of their practical nature and the requirement of simulated patients, videos and models. This book does, however, consider the likely SPs, historical scenarios and types of models and manikins, and the examination techniques that are encountered in OSCEs. Investigations and their interpretation can easily be presented in OSCE form, and candidates can expect charts, and lists of haematological and biochemical results, together with all forms of radiological investigations, with a request to interpret data and radiological abnormalities.

OSCE stations are suitable for most aspects of treatment and prognosis. It is essential to remember that treatment of a 'medical' illness should not be limited to drugs or that of a 'surgical' illness to surgery alone. They should include all forms of available and desirable intervention. This avoids the 'pigeon-holing' of disease entities into conventional specialities which is deprecated in current clinical teaching. Counselling skills and the assessment of ethical factors in clinical practice are readily tested in an OSCE setting as SPs can provide both the background and the patient's attitude to an illness. The practical application of clinical skills and procedures are also readily assessed, usually with the aid of a manikin which allows such procedures as venous catheterization, cardiopulmonary resuscitation, securing and maintaining an air-way, wound debridement and suturing.

Desirable Features of OSCEs

OSCEs bring a new dimension to the assessment of medical training. Of particular value is their ability to examine practical and other skills in a unified, measurable and reproducible fashion. This is in keeping with current trends towards performance based assessment throughout health care. OSCEs provide for an effective use of the examination time, examiners' time and commitment. They are effective in assessing knowledge and practical skills and ensure that each student is presented with the same material, thus providing a uniform evaluation with consistent marking of all those involved.

The validity of the response to each question is primarily related to the student's ability: in well constructed questions, very little variation is dependent on the examiner's responses in manned stations. The reliability of OSCEs in differentiating good from bad students and the inter-rater reliability of examiners is good, and becomes increasingly certain as the number of stations devoted to each component part is increased. Both construct and content validity have been well established.

Well constructed questions are durable and can stand up to repeated use without weakening their value. Like many forms of assessment, effective questions represent the core curriculum material, and once a suitable bank size has been achieved, security of the questions is unnecessary as knowledge of the answers represents a passable understanding of the curriculum. Experiments on presenting a single station at a time to groups of students have not reduced their value in differentiating clinical performance. Assessment can be by the students themselves or by peer review. This modification substantially reduces the necessary space and organisation for an OSCE.

OSCEs can be a useful teaching modality. With the reduced stay of patients in hospitals and increased community-based education, medical schools often have to extend their teaching practice onto a number of sites. All these factors increase the need for uniformity of teaching methods as well as assessment. This can be effectively achieved with the use of OSCEs, and the reduced number of available patients can be addressed by the use of standard patients with good effect. One well-proven example of the use of simulated patients has been in the training and assessment of trauma, linked to the Advanced Trauma Life Support and related programmes. The use of students as SPs has proved an important and enjoyable learning experience, as well as, in some cases, providing financial rewards.

- Construct validity is the ability of the OSCE to differentiate students' ability, or to follow a student's progress before and after a course of instruction.
- Content (criterion-based) validity assesses the value of the station in reaching its specified objective. In all these measures OSCEs have proved effective in student assessment and are accepted by staff and students as a fair and desirable form of assessment.

Assessment is a powerful learning tool and should be used as part of the teaching and learning processes but it must be accompanied by adequate feedback in order to benefit individual students. This process should also be used in auditing teaching methods and to stimulate any necessary changes. It is feasible to set up OSCEs in any medical school, provided appropriate staff time is allowed for their introduction. Some schools involve students in the design and development of OSCEs and it can increase their awareness of this form of assessment. The formulation of OSCEs should be closely linked with curriculum development and keyed into the curriculum objectives.

When using OSCEs to evaluate teaching methods, two types of error should be considered.

- Type I errors are those of fact, implying a deficiency of teaching and/or learning, reflecting omissions and ineffective or absent experience.
- Type II errors are defects of understanding, where a student fails to recognise or interpret a clinical situation. This reflects poor concept attainment and an inability to discriminate.

Locating these errors points to the direction that future teaching should follow.

Disadvantages of OSCEs

As discussed in the previous section, the value of OSCEs in training and assessment has been demonstrated in many fields and many such assessment packages are available. However, medical schools should not become involved in this form of assessment without allowing adequate staff time for their development and OSCEs should not become the only form of assessment.

The preparation of OSCEs requires a good deal of thought and time. The whole staff should be aware of, and preferably involved in, their development and students should have experience prior to any examination so that they can be comfortable with this form of assessment. An OSCE requires a great deal of organisation in collecting material, appropriate patients, laying out stations and making sure staff are available for manned areas. Setting up the examination can be costly on administration and on medical staff and patients, and includes the hidden costs of Faculty time in the development of the exercise.

Analysis of the data and ensuring the validity of the examination requires painstaking activity. The weighting of key questions on essential knowledge has to be resolved before any feedback to staff or students. Standard setting should be based on expected knowledge and the skills required and this relies as much on that much-criticized 'gut feeling' as it does on statistical formulae. Standardised patients, both actual and simulated have to be found and trained and an adequate pool must be available to cover expected needs. When introducing OSCEs, a school has to decide whether it is as an additional assessment or whether it should replace a previous part of the examination. If the latter, it is essential that other important areas are not diluted in the process. OSCEs are not ideal in assessing interpersonal skills: video clips or trained patients can be rather artificial in this respect. For patient examination, OSCEs do not provide a comprehensive evaluation of all aspects of a learning and educational programme and therefore should be part of a multi-component assessment in the final examination, forming a useful means of determining practical skills over a wide area.

In spite of their potential limitations, OSCEs do provide a valuable addition to the clinical exit examination and students and staff should become well acquainted with their format and appreciate their discriminatory properties.

How to Use this Book

This book contains a series of OSCE questions. The chapters are arranged by organ system, and every chapter follows the same organisation of questions, i.e. history, examination, investigation, treatment, practical techniques and other issues. The second half of the book provides the answers, together with teaching notes and a marking scheme. There is no index but the contents list will direct you to the appropriate organ system.

In the history and counselling stations, you are advised to work with one to two colleagues to act as 'patient' and 'examiner'. The Introduction provides the background required to direct your enquiry or your counselling. Take a history from the 'patient', who will answer your questions using the history provided. The 'examiner' will mark your answers, using the scoring system outlines below, and ensure that the station is concluded in the allotted time.

The clinical examination stations include clinical photographs and test clinical skills which can be practised on appropriate patients on the ward. As the practical skills of examination cannot be assessed by a text book, a check list is included, indicating what the examiner is looking for in your examination of each system. The radiographic questions may be self-assessed by turning to the answer section.

Stations with radiographs or photographs may also carry statements requiring a 'true' or 'false' response. This adds variety to the station format and requires you to assess the answers given with respect to the radiograph or photograph. Similarly, stations with tables depicting clinical scenarios or treatment regimes test your knowledge in rearranging the latter to fit the disease.

At the back of the book there is a section that explains the marking schedule used for the stations, and a mock exam that contains five 19-station OSCE circuits: these provide typical examination scenarios.

By working through each organ system, as denoted by the chapters, you will cover most of the OSCE station scenarios and variations that you can expect to encounter in the undergraduate course.

Scoring your performance

We have chosen not to weight individual questions or items. Good is allocated 3 marks and adequate 2. In the poor/not done column the assessor can differentiate between a reasonable but inadequate mark and poor or not done. This differentiation can direct future study requirements. Each station is allocated the same mark, item scores are added in three column answers. Two of three correct responses or a mean score of 2 is a pass. A 60% correct response rate is required in two column answers. In the mock examinations two-thirds of stations should be passed to pass the examination.

Glossary

A-level	Advanced Level General Certificate of Education – School leaving Examination
ABGs	Arterial blood gases
AC	Abdominal circumference
ACE inhibitors	Angiotensin converting enzyme
ACTH	Adrenocorticotrophic hormone
Ach	Acetylcholine
ACS	Acute coronary syndrome
ADH	Anti-diuretic hormone
ADL	Activity of daily living
AF	Atrial fibrilation
AFP	Alpha-fetoprotein
aGBM	Anti-glomerular basement membrane
AGT	Angiotensin
AIDS	Acquired immune deficiency syndrome
AKA	Also known as
Alb	Albumin
Alk phos	Alkaline phosphatase
ALT	Alanine amino-transferase
AMA	Antimitochondrial antibody
ANCA	Anti neutrophil cytoplasmic antibody
Anti dsDNA	Double stranded deoxyribonucleic acid
Anti-Jo	Specific antigen
Anti-La	Specific antigen
Anti-RNP	Ribonucleic protein
Anti-Ro	Specific antigen
Anti-SCL70	Specific antigen
AP	Antero-posterior
APC gene	Adenomatosis polyposis coli
APTT	Activated partial thromboplastin time
ARDS	Adult respiratory distress syndrome
ARM	Artificial rupture of membranes
AS	Aortic stenosis
ASH	Action on smoking and health
ASMA	anti- smooth muscle antibody
ASO(T)	Anti streptolysin-O-titre
AST	Aspartate amino-transferase
ATLS	Advanced trauma life support
AV	Arterio-venous

AV	Atrio-ventricular
aVF	Augmented voltage lead left lower leg
aVL	Augmented voltage lead left arm
aVR	Augmented voltage lead right arm
AVSD	Atrioventricular septal defect
AXR	Abdominal X-ray
AZT	Azidothymidine (Generic Name: Zidovudine)
BAL	Broncho-alveolar lavage
BBB	Bundle branch block
BCC	Basal cell carcinoma
BCG	Bacille Calmette-Guerin
b.d.	Bis die (twice daily)
BE	Base excess
BHL	Bilateral hilar lymphadenopathy
BMA	British Medical Association
BM stix	Blood monitoring
BM	Bone marrow
BMI	Body mass index
BMR	Basal metabolic rate
BP	Blood pressure
Bpm	Beats per minute
BRCA	Breast cancer susceptibility genes
C	Cervical
Ca	Cancer
CA	Cyclic AMP
$Ca2+$	Calcium
CAGE questionnaire	Cut down Annoyed Guilty Eye-opener
CANCA	Anti-neutrophil cytoplasmic antibody
CAPD	Chronic ambulatory peritoneal dialysis
CCa^{2+}	Corrected calcium
CD4	A surface antigen principally found on helper-inducer T-lymphocyte
CEA	Carcinoembryonic antigen
CEMD	Confidential Enquiry into Maternal Health
CESDI	Confidential Enquiry into Stillbirths and Deaths in Infancy
CF	Cystic fibrosis
CIN I II III	Cervical intraepithelial neoplasia
CK	Creatinine phosphokinase
Cl	Chloride
CLL	Chronic lymphocytic leukaemia
Cm	Centimetre
CML	Chronic myeloid leukaemia

CMV	Cytomegalovirus
CNS	Central nervous system
CO2	Carbon dioxide
COCP	Combined oral contraceptive pill
COMT	Catechol O-methyl transferase
CPN	Community psychiatric nurse
CPR	Cardio pulmonary resuscitation
Cr	Creatinine
CREST	Crest syndrome – calcinosis; Raynaud's; oesophageal dysmotility; sclerodactyly; telangiectasia
CS	Caesarean section
CSF	Cerebro-spinal fluid
CSU	Catheter specimen of urine
CT	Computerised tomography
CTG	Cardiotocography
CVA	Cerebro-vascular accident
CVP	Central venous pressure
CVS	Chorionic villi sampling
CWD	Consistent with dates
CXR	Chest radiograph
DDAVP	Desmopressin, synthetic vasopressin
DIC	Disseminated intravascular coagulopathy
DIP joints	Distal inter-phalangeal joints
DKA	Diabetic keto-acidosis
dl	Decilitres
DM	Diabetes mellitus
DMSA	Dimercaptosuccinic acid
DNA	Deoxyribonucleic acid
DTP	Diphtheria-tetanus pertussis (vaccine)
DU	Duodenal ulcer
DVT	Deep vein thrombosis
DVLA	Driving vehicle licensing authority
ECG	Electrocardiogram
EEG	Electroencephalogram
EMQ	Extended matching question
ENT	Ear, nose and throat
ERCP	Endoscopic retrograde cholangiopancreatography
ESR	Erythrocyte sedimentation rate
ETEC	Enterotoxigenic Escherichia coli
EUA	Examination under anaestesia
FBC	Full blood count
FEV1	Forced expiratory volume in one second

FFP	Fresh frozen plasma
FH	Family history
5-FU	5-Fluoro-uracil
5HT	5-hydroxy-tryptamine
fl	Femtolitres
F:M	Female:male (ratio)
FNA	Fine needle aspirate
FPC	Family planning clinic
FSH	Follicular stimulating hormone
fT4	Free thyroxine
FVC	Forced vital capacity
GABA	Gamma- amino butyric acid
GCS	Glasgow coma score
GCSE	General Certificate of Secondary Education
GCSF	Granulocyte colony stimulating factor
GDM	Gestational diabetes mellitus
GI	Gastrointestinal
GIT	Gastrointestinal tract
GMC	General Medical Council
GnRH	Gonadotrophin-releasing hormone
GP	General Practitioner
GPI	General paralysis of the insane
G6PD	Glucosa 6 phosphate dehydrogenase
GTN	Glyceryl trinitrate
GIIb/IIIa	Glycoprotein IIb/IIIa (receptor)
GU	Genito-urinary
GUM	Genito-urinary medicine
Hb	Haemoglobin
HB Alc	Glycosylated haemoglobin
HBV	Hepatitis B virus
HCG	Human chorionic gonadotrophin
HCO3–	Bicarbonate
Hct–	Haematocrit
HCV	Hepatitis C virus
HDL	High density lipoprotein
HELLP	Elevated liver enzymes and low platelet count
HIB	*Haemophilus influenzae* type B (vaccine)
HIV	Human immunodeficiency virus
HLA	Human leucocyte antigen
HONK	Hyper-osmolar non-ketotic (coma)
HR	Heart rate
HRT	Hormaone replacement therapy

HSV	Herpes simplex virus
IBD	Inflammatory bowel disease
ICP	Intra-cranial pressure
IDDM	Insulin dependent diabetes mellitus
Ig	Immunoglobulin
IgM	Immunoglobulin M
IGT	Impaired glucose tolerance
IHD	Ischaemic heart disease
Im	Intramuscular
IMB	Intermenstrual bleeding
INR	International ratio
IOL	Induction of labour
IQ	Intelligence quotient
ISMN	Iso-sorbide mono-nitrate
ITU	Intensive therapy unit
IUCD	Intrauterine contraceptive device
IUGR	Intrauterine growth retardation
IV	Intravenous
IVP	Intravenous pyelogram
IVF	Invitro fertilisation
IVU	Intravenous urogram
K^+	Potassium
Kg	Kilogramme
KPa	Kilopascals
KUB	Kidneys/ureters/bladder
L	Litre
LDL	Low density lipoprotein
LFT	Liver function tests
LGV	Lymphogranuloma venereum
LH	Luteinising hormone
LHRH	Luteinising hormone releasing hormone
LKM-1	Liver, kidney, Muscle
LLETZ	Large Loop Excision of the Transformation Zone
LMN	Lower motor neurone
LMW	Low molecular weight
LNMP	Last normal menstrual period
LSCS	Lower segment caesarean section
MAOI	Mono-amine oxidase inhibitor
MCH	Mean corpuscular haemoglobin
MCP	Meta-carpophalangeal
MCV	Mean corpuscular volume
Mg^{++}	Magnesium

MI	Myocardial infarction
mmol	Millimoles
MMR	Measles-mumps-rubella (vaccine)
MMSE	Mini mental state examination
Mph	Miles per hour
MRI	Magnetic resonance imaging
MS	Multiple sclerosis or Mitral stenosis
MSU	Mid stream urine
Na^+	Sodium
NAD	No abnormality detected
NEC	Necrotising enterocolitis
Neut	Neutrophilis
NG	Neoplasia (new growth)
NHL	Non-Hodgkin's lymphoma
NIDDM	Non insulin dependent diabetes mellitus
NSAID	Non steroidal anti-inflammatory drug
NSU	Non-specific urethritis
O2	Oxygen
OA	Osteoarthritis
OCP	Oral contraceptive pill
Od	Omni die (once daily)
OGD	Oesophagogastroduodenoscopy
OSCE	Objective structured clinical examination
PA	Postero-anterior
$PaCO_2$	Arterial pressure of carbon dioxide
PaO_2	Arterial pressure of oxygen
PAN	Perinuclear anti-neutrophilic
Panca	Perinuclear anti-neutrophilic cytoplasmic antibody
PCO	Polycystic ovaries
PCOS	Polycystic ovary syndrome
PCP	Pneumocystis carinii pneumonia
PCR	Polymerase chain reaction
PCV	Packed cell volume
PDA	Patent ductus arteriosus
PE	Pulmonary embolism
PEA	Persistent electrical activity
PEFR	Peak expiratory flow rate
PET	positron emission tomography
pH	Puissance d'Hydrogen = $- \log (H+)$
PICU	Paediatric intensive care unit
PID	Pelvic inflammatory disease
Plats	Platelets

PMH	Previous medical history
PND	Paroxysmal nocturnal dyspnoea
PNS	Peripheral nervous system
PO4⁻	Phosphate
PPH	Post partum haemorrhage
PPI	Proton pump inhibitor
PR	Per rectum
PRHO	Pre-registration house officer
PRN	Pro re nata (as required)
PSA	Prostatic specific antigen
PT	Prothrombin time
PV	Per vagina
RBC	Red blood count
RCT	Randomised, controlled trial
Retics	Reticulocytes
ROM	Range of movement
RTA	Road traffic accident
RTA (I–IV)	Renal tubular acidosis
SACD	Subacute combined degeneration of the spinal cord
SAH	Subarachnoid haemorrhage
SARS	Severe acute respiratory syndrome
SCC	Squamous cell carcinoma
SDH	Subdural haemorrhage
SHBG	Sex hormone binding globulin
SIADH	Syndrome of inappropriate antidiuretic hormone secretion
SLE	Systemic lupus erythema
SOL	Space occupying lesion
SROM	spontaneous rupture of membranes
SSRI	Selective serotonin reuptake inhibitors
STEMI	ST elevation MI
STI	Sexually transmitted disease
Substance P	Vasoactive peptide and sensory neurotransmitter found in nerve cells and specialist gut endocrine cells SVT Supraventricular tachycardia
SVD	Spontaneous vaginal delivery
SVT	Supraventricular tachycardia
SXR	Skull X-ray
T3	Tri-iodo – thyronine
T4	Tetra – iodo -thyronine (thyroxine)
TB	Tuberculosis
TBM	Tuberculous meningitis
Tds	Ter die sumendus – (to be taken three times daily)

TED	Thrombo-embolic
TFTs	Thyroid function tests
T Helper	Thymus (lymphocytes)
TKco	Transfer coefficient
TIA	Transient ischaemic attack
TOP	Termination of pregnancy
TPA	Tissue plasminogen activator
TPHA	Treponema pallidum haemagglutination assay
TSH	Thyroid stimulating hormone
TT	Thrombin time
TVM	Transvaginal monitoring
U&Es	Urea and electrolytes
UMN	Upper motor neurone
Ur	Urea
USS	Ultrasound scan
UTI	Urinary tract infection
UV	Ultra violet
UV prolapse	Utero-vaginal prolapse
VDRL	Venereal disease research laboratory
VMA	Vanillylmandelic acid
V/Q scan	Ventilation/perfusion scan
VSD	Ventricular septal defect
V-V Fistula	Vesico-vaginal fistula
VZV	Varicella zoster virus
WCC	White cell count

Normal Values

In the majority of OSCE data interpretation stations it is customary in undergraduate examination to provide a set of normal values. Please refer to the list below when attempting any of the data interpretation stations in all three volumes of OSCEs.

Haematology

Haemoglobin		
	Males	13.5 – 17.5 g/dl
	Females	11.5 – 15.5 g/dl
MCV		76 – 98 fl
PCV		35 – 55%
WCC		4 – 11 x 10^9/l
Neut.		2.5 – 7.58 x 10^9/l
Lymph.		1.5 – 3.5 x 10^9/l
Plt		150 – 400 x 10^9/l
ESR		0 – 10 mm in the 1st hour
PT		10.6 – 14.9 s
PTT		23.0 – 35.0 s
TT		10.5 – 15.5 s
Fib		125 – 300 mg/dl
Vitamin B$_{12}$		160 – 900 pmol/l
Folate		1.5 µg/l
Ferritin		
	Males	20 – 250 µmol/l
	Females	10 – 120 µmol/l

Immunoglobulins

IgM	0.5 – 2.0 g/l
IgG	5 – 16 g/l
IgA	1.0 – 4.0 g/l

Biochemistry

Na$^+$	135 – 145 mmol/l
K$^+$	3.5 – 5.0 mmol/l
Urea (ur)	2.5 – 6.5 mmol/l
Cr	50 – 120 µmol/l
ALT	5 – 30 Iu/l
AST	10 – 40 iu/l
Bili.	2 – 17 µmol/l
Alk Phos	30 – 130 iu/l
Albumin	35 – 55 g/l
γGT	5 – 30 iu/l

αFP   < 10 ku/l
CCA^{2+} 2.20 – 2.60 mmol/l
PO$_4$$^{2-}$ 0.70 – 1.40 mmol/l
CK   23 – 175 iu/l
LDH   100 – 190 iu/l
Amylase   < 200 u/l
Lactate   0.5 – 2.2 mmol/l
Mg^{2+} 0.75 – 1.00 mmol/l
Urate   0.1 – 0.4 mol/l
CRP   0 – 10 mg/l

Diabetes
Glucose

    Random   3.5 – 5.5 mmol/l*
    Fasting   < 7 mmol/l
HbA1c   < 7.0%

Endocrinology
TSH   0.17 – 3.2 mu/l
fT$_4$ 11 – 22 pmol/l
fT$_3$ 3.5 – 5 pmol/l
Cortisol

    0900   140 – 500 nmol/l
    2400   50 – 300 nmol/l
Growth hormone   < 10 ng/ml
Cholesterol   < 5.2 mmol/l
Triglycerides   0 – 1.5 mmol/l
LDL   < 3.5 mmol/l
HDL   > 1.0 mmol/l
Total/ HDL   < 5.0
FSH   1 – 25 u/l
LH   1 – 70 u/l
Prolactin   < 400 mu/l

Blood gases
pH   7.35 – 7.45
pA (CO_2)   4.6 – 6.0 kPa
pA (CO_2)   10.5 – 13.5 kPa
HCO$_3$$^-$ (bicarbonate) 24 – 30 mmol/l
BE   −2 – 2.0 mmol/l

CSF

Protein	< 0.45 g/l
Glucose	2.5 – 3.9 mmol/l (two-thirds plasma)
Cells	< 5 (WCC)
Opening pressure	6 – 20 cmH$_2$O

* If >5.5 then OGTT 2 h: 7 – 11.1 = IGT

           > 11.1 = DM

Generic approach to examinations

As with all OSCE stations, clinical examination stations should have clear, precise candidate instructions. **Read them carefully before starting** (and before asking any questions!) and if you are still unclear as to what you are being asked to do, clarify the task with the examiner.

For all clinical examinations you should try and follow the five steps given below. Some examinations may require you to modify or vary these stages:

1 **Introduction and consent**
2 **Observation and comment**
3 **Palpation**
4 **Auscultation**
5 **Presentation of findings and differential diagnoses or causes**

1 Introduction and consent

- Introduce yourself to the patient: with your name and role
- Explain what you would like to do and obtain verbal consent for the examination, eg 'I am just going to listen to your heart sounds, 'is that alright?' or 'Would it be alright if I examine your chest, legs'
- Keep these requests simple and in lay terms. Avoid medical jargon such as 'I would like to examine your peripheral nervous system' or 'would it be alright if I examine your cranial nerves?' Better to ask 'Would it be alright if I examine the function of your arms or legs' or ' Would it be alright if I examine the function of the nerves that control your face?'

2 Observation and comment

- Stand at the **END** of the patient's bed and comment on relative positives and negative manifestations. Look for relevant signs and they will be there – If you fail to look for them, they may not appear!
- Do not just say 'I'm looking for...'. **Comment** on the presence or absence of relevant signs
- Move back to the patient's right-hand side, re-clarify before starting your examination if you should start at the hands (if not stated in the instructions)
- **Look** for relevant signs – **comment** on their presence/absence.
- BUT expect to be challenged on findings/causes of anything you mention.

3 Palpation

- Be sure you have washed your hands in warm water before commencing any the examination. There is usually an alcohol wash at the bedside of each patient, which you should use between stations. If not, you should wash your hands between each patient, but be careful you do not leave the examiner behind, as he or she might be a little irritated.
- Whenever palpating:
  - (i)   Reassure the patient before starting
  - (ii) Watch the patient's face for distress at all times
  - (iii) Apologise if any distress is caused
  - (iv) If distressed before the start of the examination – suggest appropriate analgesia.

4 Auscultation

- Understand what the stethoscope and its components are for, ie how to use the bell and the diaphragm (Bell = Low frequency) and even which way round to put the earpieces in your ears!
- Always tap the piece (bell or diaphragm) you are about to place on the patient with a finger, thus ensuring it is orientated the correct way. This saves 'no sounds heard': embarrassing silence!
- Always make sure the stethoscope pieces are warm (like you hands) before placing them on the patient.
- Your stethoscope should hang so the bell/diaphragm lies just below your waistline. This means you may need to cut longer tubes down but be wary of cutting off too much!
- With the more expensive/sophisticated stethoscopes you will hear sounds more easily and clearly. However, you may wish to buy a mid range one first to learn the basics.
- Know how to use the stethoscope, if you choose to buy an expensive/sophisticated one.

As with all the examination techniques, palpation, ballotting, auscultation and percussion, practice makes perfect! Initially you may feel more comfortable practising in the clinical skills laboratory on manikins and normal people, however **you must** practice in the various clinical settings on patients with and without clinical signs. Essential parts of the examination cannot be practised on friends and mannequins. Overcoming embarrassment or anxieties, talking and interacting with patients and relatives and, most importantly, recognising when patients are ill and eliciting clinical signs. At the end of every examination make sure you cover the patient up and thank them. Take every opportunity to examine patients, checking appropriate subjects with housemen and your peers, but make sure you have permission from the patient and the sister-in-charge.

5 Presentation of clinical findings, differential diagnoses and causes.

- Your presentation should be simple and concise. Present relevant positives and negatives, a differential diagnosis or causes.
- If you know the diagnosis, present the positive findings to support your diagnosis.
- 'This well looking, middle-aged man has signs consistent with aortic stenosis as evidenced by his low volume pulse which was slow rising in character. He has a narrow pulse pressure and his apex beat is hyperdynamic but undisplaced. On auscultation he has a grade 4/6 ejection systolic murmur heard loudest in the aortic area and radiating to the carotids. He has no signs of heart failure and no stigmata of endocarditis'.
- If you do not know the diagnosis, present the relevant positive and negative findings in a concise, logical manner. The simplest way to achieve this is to present the evaluations in the order of your examination, ie start at the hands, work up the forearm, the arm (including blood pressure), the face and neck, chest, abdomen and other regions of interest.
- 'This well looking middle-aged man had no peripheral stigmata of cardiovascular disease. His pulse was 72 bpm and regular, it was symmetrical and I was unsure but I think the character was abnormal. His blood pressure was 110/100 but I couldn't see his jugular venous pulse. His carotids were easily felt and had an abnormal character, although I couldn't define it. The apex beat was undisplaced and forceful. He had no heaves or thrills. On auscultation he had a systolic murmur heard loudest in the aortic area and I think it radiated to the carotids and the mitral area. He had no pulmonary or peripheral oedema. In summary, I think he may have aortic stenosis'.
- At the end of your presentation you should present a list of the common differentials or causes of the patient's problem.
- The examiner may challenge you on anything that you state, eg if you say the patient has clubbing, you might be asked some causes of clubbing.
- As with all clinical skills, presentation of findings and differentials requires practice.

Chapter 1:
Gastroenterology

Contents

Gastroenterology and Hepatobiliary Disease – History

Gastroenterology and Hepatobiliary Disease – Examination

Chapter 1

Gastroenterology

Gastroenterology and Hepatobiliary Disease – History

Diarrhoea

- **Age of the patient:**
  Under 40 – think irritable bowel disease, infective, irritable bowel
  Over 40 – think carcinoma
- **Duration of the illness** – 'when were you last well?'

What does the patient mean by diarrhoea?
Increased frequency
Increased volume of stool

- **Frequency**
  How many times in a 24 hour period is the patient opening their bowels?
  Do they have to get up at night to defecate?

- **Consistency of the stools**
  Watery/clear/frothy
  Fluid/brown
  Semiformed
  Solid
  Presence or absence of blood
  Presence or absence of mucus
  Steatorrhoea-like stool
  Pale, offensive, porridge like stools which float in the toilet water and are difficult to flush away

Features associated with diarrhoea
- Systemic signs and symptoms: anaemia pyrexia, arthritis, sacroiliitis, uveitis, erythema nodosum
- Nausea and vomiting; dehydration
- Abdominal pain: character, site, radiation, relief, exacerbation
- Weight loss, loss of appetite (anorexia)
- Recent foreign travel, particularly to epi/endemic areas
- Family history of inflammatory bowel disease, bowel polyps/cancer

Differential diagnoses

The main causes of diarrhoea are colonic. Small bowel causes are rare

- **Colonic causes**

   Inflammatory bowel disease

   Infective colitis

     Bacterial:

     E. Coli, Salmonella typhi and *paratyphi*

     Campylobacter, Shigella, Yersinia, *Vibrio cholerae,*

     Clostridium difficile

     Viral: rotavirus, adenovirus, astrovirus

     Protozoal: *Giardia lamblia, Entamoeba histolytica*, Cryptosporidium (in the immunosuppressed)

Left-sided colonic malignancy

Ischaemic colitis

Overflow diarrhoea secondary to constipation

- **Small bowel causes**

   Coeliac disease

   Secretory or high output diarrhoea, eg post small bowel resection

   VIPoma

   Terminal ileitis, eg TB or Crohn's disease

Bleeding per rectum

History

- 'Spotting' and fresh blood stains on toilet tissue during or following bowel action: found in haemorrhoids or fissure
- Fresh and/or profuse bleeding (egg cupful or more): found in diverticular disease, inflammatory bowel disease, arterio-venous malformation or carcinoma
- Dark/altered blood: usually from lesions in the proximal colon (diverticular disease or carcinoma) or rarely small bowel
- 'Red currant jelly' stool: intussusception in children
- Mucoid bloody diarrhoea: in enteric infections such as typhoid and amoebiasis

Associated features

- Altered bowel habits: loose motions alternating with constipation
- Mucus in stool
- Abdominal pain/discomfort, abdominal mass
- Tenesmus
- Weight loss

Causes

- Piles and fissures: commonest cause in adults (may present as a 'red herring' masking a bowel tumour)
- Diverticular disease: commonest cause in middle age and the elderly
- Colonic carcinoma: must be excluded by colonoscopy or bowel imaging
- Anal carcinoma: uncommon, palpable on digital examination

Upper GI bleed

History

- Haematemesis: fresh blood, altered blood or coffee grounds
- Volume of vomitus and amount of blood
- How many episodes/volume of each episode at this presentation
- Passage of melaena
- Previous episodes/causes if known

Associated features

- Epigastric pain – acute/chronic, character, radiation, relief, exacerbation
- Epigastric fullness, weight loss, anorexia
- Dyspepsia
- Features of chronic liver disease

Risk factors

- Use of NSAIDs – duration
- Other medications: steroids, anticoagulants
- Known or previous peptic ulcer disease, varices or hiatus hernia
- Alcohol excess: duration, amount, type of alcohol
- Chronic liver disease
- Familial blood dyscrasia

Causes

In anatomical sequence:

- Oesophageal: oesophagitis, carcinoma, varices, Mallory–Weiss tear, trauma, hiatus hernia
- Gastric: gastritis, peptic ulcer, benign and malignant tumours, eg leiomyoma, adenocarcinoma
- Duodenal: duodenitis, peptic ulcer

Dysphagia

- Level of the dysphagia: oropharynx; high, mid or lower oesophagus
- Degree of dysphagia: solids, semi-solids, liquids
- Progression: insidious, intermittent onset signifies benign disease; a rapidly progressive course implies malignancy
- Pain: suggests local inflammatory process or infection, eg candidiasis 'Impaction pain' is typical of benign stricturing
- Regurgitation: immediate/delayed

Associated features

- Weight loss, anorexia
- Features of systemic diseases:
  Raynaud's (systemic sclerosis)
  Muscle weakness and wasting (motor neurone disease)
  Ptosis (myasthenia gravis)
- Change in bowel habit
- Coughing/recurrent chest infection – implies aspiration

Causes

- Oropharynx
  Bulbar palsy, eg motor neurone disease, myasthenia gravis
  tonsilitis, pharyngeal pouch
- Oesophageal
  Benign stricture: gastro-oesophageal reflux; corrosives
  Malignant stricture: upper oesophagus – squamous carcinoma;
  lower oesophagus – adenocarcinoma
- Hiatus hernia
- Infective: candidiasis, CMV, HSV (particularly in HIV disease)
- Chagas' disease (South American trypanosomiasis)
- Oesophageal web (Plummer–Vinson or Paterson–Brown Kelly syndrome)
- Extrinsic compression eg bronchial carcinoma, left atrial hypertrophy, retrosternal goitre, mediastinal lymphadenopathy

Risk factors for oesophageal carcinoma:

- Smoking
- Alcohol excess
- Possible dietary factors (nitrosamines in diet)
- Achalasia of the cardia
- Plummer–Vinson syndrome
- Tylosis

Jaundice

Causes

* Pre-hepatic – haemolysis
* Hepatic – cirrhosis, infective hepatitis, drugs
* Obstructive – gallstones, carcinoma of the gall bladder, pancreas, ampulla of Vater, pancreatitis, biliary stricture

Differentiating questions

* Alcohol consumption
* Travel abroad
* Family history
* Recreational drug use
* Previous jaundice/cause
* Weight loss
* Food Poisoning

* Previous blood transfusions
* Recent contacts
* Sexual contacts
* Medications
* Fever/viral prodrome
* Dark urine/pale stools – signs of obstructive disease

Differentiating acute and chronic liver disease

* On examination of jaundiced patients it is important to differentiate between acute and acute on chronic liver disease. One must therefore look for signs of chronic liver disease
* Hands: clubbing, leuconychia, palmar erythema, Dupuytren's contracture
* Upper limbs: scratch marks, bruising
* Chest: gynaecomastia, loss of male distribution of hair, spider naevi
* Abdomen: hepatosplenomegaly, ascites, caput medusae, gonadal atrophy
* Confusion, hepatic fetor and liver flap are signs of hepatic encephalopathy

Gastroenterology and Hepatobiliary Disease – Examination

Introduction

Many patients with abdominal pathology present with abdominal pain. The characteristics of the pain including site, character, radiation, exacerbating and relieving factors and associated features such as jaundice, dysphagia, diarrhoea, constipation and abdominal distention all help in the differential diagnoses and direct the clinical examination and subsequent investigations. Abdominal pain may be acute or chronic and in the acute cases, severity of the pain and the accompanying peritonism, are important factors in determining the need for urgent surgical or other intervention. Such emergencies require the patient to remain nil by mouth with passage of a nasogastric tube if there is nausea or distention, and intravenous fluids in the presence of dehydration, shock or suspected blood loss.

Examination

As with all clinical examinations introduce yourself and explain the examination, gaining verbal consent to proceed. The patient traditionally is exposed from 'nipples to knees' – which implies the whole of the abdomen from above the xiphisternum to below the genitalia and inguinal regions. In clinical exams it is sufficient to expose the patient from the xiphisternum to the pubis, the inguinal region and external genitalia being examined at the end of the examination if the examiner wishes. Examination of the groins is important to identify inguinal and femoral herniae and exclude inguinal lymphadenopathy. This part of the examination should be carried out without embarrassment to patient or attendees.

Once the patient is comfortably positioned and correctly exposed:

1 Observation
At the end of the bed – look for and comment on the presence or absence of:

- Distress; well or unwell; jaundice; signs of chronic liver disease
- Abdominal distension; asymmetry; scars; masses; organomegaly

You may ask the patient to:

- draw their knees up to relax the abdomen
- take a deep inspiration observing for equal painless movement, and hepatosplenomegaly and masses

Return to the right-hand side of the patient

From the hands – look for:
Hands (clubbing, leuconychia, koilonychia, palmar erythema, Dupytren's contracture, hepatic flap)

Upper limbs (tattoos, bruising, purpura, spider naevi)
↓
Face (jaundice, xanthelasma, hepatic fetor, anaemia, dentition and ulceration of the buccal mucosa)
↓
Neck (supraclavicular lymphadenopathy – particularly a left-sided supraclavicular fossa node: Virchow's node/Trossier's sign)
↓
Chest (spider naevi, gynaecomastia, loss of male distribution of hair)
↓
Abdomen (asymmetry, scars, distention, masses, organomegaly)

2 Palpation
Always check if patient has any pain and if it is localised to any particular area of the abdomen. Try to start on the opposite side of the abdomen.

- Kneel on the right side of the patient so that you are level with the abdomen; this also stops you placing too much downwards pressure while palpating (which one tends to do if standing). Shorter people should use their common sense!
- Always warm your hands prior to placing them on the abdomen
- Throughout the examination observe the patient's face for distress
- If the patient has signs of peritonism one should check for **rebound tenderness** and **guarding**

OSCE Stations

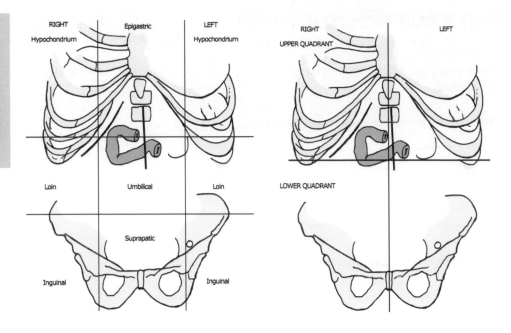

fig 1a the four quadrants of the abdomen

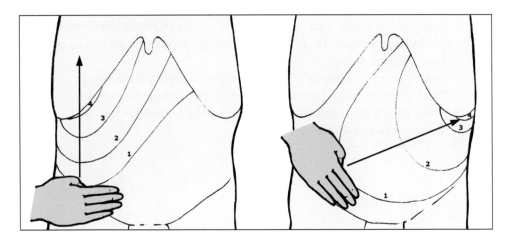

fig 1b

When examining the abdomen you should:

1 Start in the diagonally opposite side area if there is any localised area of pain
2 Examine from your MCP joints (not bending the IP joints) of the fingers
3 Examine all four quadrants of all nine areas – ie thoroughly cover the whole surface in a systematic manner

OSCE Stations

(a) Examine for the enlarged liver – see fig 1a

- Start in the right iliac fossa. At position (1) ask patient to take a deep breath in and move your hand 'up' to meet the 'descending' liver edge.
- As the patient breathes out – take your hand off and replace in position (2) – repeat process as for (1)
- Repeat in positions (3) and (4)
- Percuss and define the upper and lower borders of the liver

Positions (1)–(4) are not randomly chosen, they represent the four clinical 'enlargements' of the liver and equally in the description below the spleen, ie (1) 'giant', (2) grossly enlarged, (3) enlarged, and (4) just palpable below the costal margin. It is traditional to describe the enlargement of both liver and spleen in terms of 'finger breadths' below the costal margins, one finger breadth being approximately equal to one centimetre.

(b) Examine for the enlarged spleen – see fig 1b

Start in the right iliac fossa

- Ask the patient to take a deep breath in. Move your hand 'up' (across diagonally up towards the left costal margin) with the left hand supporting the left costal margin
- As the patient breathes out – take your hand off and replace in position (2) – then repeat (1)
- Repeat in positions (3) and (4)
- Percuss and define the upper and lower borders of the spleen

---

The five characteristics of splenomegaly – differentiating it from other left upper quadrant mass, such as a large renal mass are:

1 **You cannot get above or over it**
2 **It descends downwards and then across towards the right iliac fossa with inspiration**
3 **It is dull to percussion**
4 **It has an anterior notch**
5 **It is not bi-manually ballotable**

Remember: a spleen just palpable below the left costal margin is at least two or three times its normal size

(c) Examine for enlarged kidneys

Over the left and right loins, 'ballot' for the left and right kidneys.
The kidneys are retroperitoneal so they normally have the following characteristics
(as compared to the spleen):

- They are ballotable
- They don't move with respiration
- They are resonant to percussion
- You can get above them on palpation

However large eg polycystic kidneys may break many of these 'rules'.

(d) Examine for ascites

With planted hand facing in a head to toe direction, percuss away from yourself
towards the left loin.
If an area of dullness is elicited, ask the patient to move onto their right side ie
towards you, with planted hand still over area of dullness.
Wait for 5–10 seconds – then repercuss over the area – if ascites is present, the area
will now be resonant, demonstrating 'shifting dullness'. (At this point you could also
re-palpate for splenomegaly.)

(e) Define a mass

As with any other mass, if you palpate an intra-abdominal mass you should define
the:

- **Site**
- **External features** – size (defining upper and lower borders), shape,
  surface, colour, temperature, mobility, tenderness
- **Internal features** – consistency, compressibility, reducibility, fluctuation,
  fluid thrill, expansile, pulsatile, cough impulse, discharge, transillumination,
  presence of a bruit
- **Surrounding features** – attachments to superficial and deep structures,
  invasion of local structures, related lymphadenopathy

(f) Palpate for inguinal lymph nodes

(g) Examine for inguinal hernia

A hernia is a protrusion of the abdominal contents through a deficit in the wall (internal hernias occur when a loop of gut passes through a deficit in the mesentery and the term is also used for hiatus hernia, when the stomach slides or rolls through the oesophageal opening in the diaphragm). With an external hernia, a patient usually complains of a lump, which may or may not be painful. Complications arise from a narrowed neck of the hernia contents; bulging out may become irreducible (incarcerated), producing intestinal destruction (colic, abdominal pain, vomiting, constipation and distention) and the blood supply may be compressed at the neck and contents become ischaemic (strangulation).

Hernias are common and therefore appropriate and often available for examination. It is essential that the anatomy and the technique of examination are perfected. Although it is not ideal for a single patient to be examined repeatedly in an OSCE, a number of patients can be used in series.

If the candidate has to confirm that there is a lump, one needs to define:

- Where it is situated, ie site
- Whether it is tender
- Whether it is reducible

In all hernias, ie including ones that are difficult to find or when checking the normal side, the examination is best undertaken with the patient standing as gravity tends to extrude the abdominal contents. However, if there is a large hernia or if the patient is already lying down, the initial examination is carried out in this position.

A key feature is an understanding of the anatomy of the inguinal canal, so that you can put your finger on the right spot and feel a cough impulse. Reduce the lump, then find if you can control the cough impulse by imposing pressure over the suspected neck of the sac. Figs 1c and 1d indicates the anatomy of direct and indirect inguinal and femoral herniae.

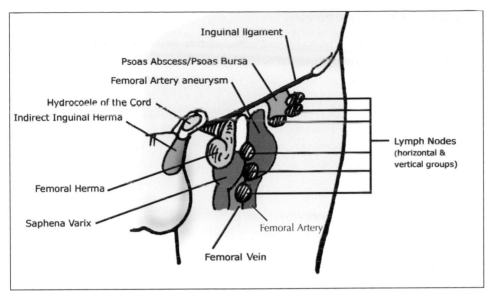

fig 1c Examining for hepatomegaly

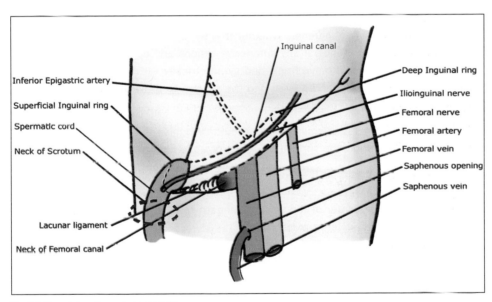

fig 1d Examining for splenomegaly

3 Auscultation

Listen for bowel sounds and bruits. Palpate femoral pulses; define abdominal aortic aneurysm (if present).

4 To complete your examination

- 'I would like to perform a per rectal (PR) examination' to assess and comment on:
  - peri-anal disease
  - rectal disease
  - prostate assessment (in men)
  - stool colour/melaena

- Examine the external genitalia
- Record temperature, BP and pulse
- Urinalsis:
  - urobilinogen
  - leucocytes; nitrites
  - haematuria
  - proteinuria

Abdominal extras

1 Inspection

Observe the shape of the abdomen, whether it is symmetrical, obese, distended, full in certain areas, the presence of any cutaneous lesions and operation or other scars. The abdominal wall should move freely and symmetrically with respiration; this can be further tested and pain noted by asking the patient to draw the abdomen in and then blow it out, followed by a cough.

Scars indicate previous problems and you should recognise the common ones as indicated in fig 00. Know the surface markings of abdominal viscera, namely:

- The upper border of the liver, in the right 4th intercostal space in the midclavicular line
- The anterior border of the spleen, beneath the 9th, 10th and 11th ribs, reaching the posterior axiliary line
- The pylorus, just to the right of the midline in the transpyloric plane (midway between the suprasternal notch and the symphysis pubis)
- The gallbladder, beneath the tip of the 9th costal cartilage
- The duodenojejunal flexure, just to the left of the midline and just below the transpyloric plane
- The base of the appendix, at the junction of the middle and lateral thirds of the line joining the ubilicus and the right anterior superior iliac spine
- The hilum of each kidney, approximately in the transpyloric plane 10 cm from the midline (the left slightly higher than the right)
- The deep inguinal ring, just above the midpoint of the inguinal ligament (passing from the anterior superior iliac spine to the pubic tubercle)

2 Palpation

Palpation determines the presence of tenderness, guarding and rigidity. Ask the patient to indicate the area of tenderness and leave examination of this area till last.

Other useful techniques for demonstrating tenderness while producing minimal discomfort are percussion rebound (see below) and asking the patient to palpate their own abdomen, to see how carefully they press in certain areas. In children, further confidence may be gained by using the child's hand underneath your own in the abdominal palpation.

Palpation commences with gentle pressure in the four quadrants, leaving the tender area till last. Once the degree of tenderness is established, deeper palpation can be undertaken, to look for abdominal masses in these areas, and up and down the midline, particularly looking for neoplasms of the stomach and pancreas, retroperitoneal masses and nodes, and aorto–iliac aneurysms.

Next palpate the liver, spleen and kidneys. For the liver, commence in the right iliac fossa, with the index finger placed transversely, moving cranially in stages. See if the edge can be palpated on deep inspiration, proceeding in four or five steps to the right costal margin. The spleen is similarly assessed from the right iliac fossa across the umbilicus to the left subcostal margin, then rolling the patient slightly onto the right side to deeply palpate beneath the costal margin in the midaxillary line, where the tip of the spleen is first felt.

The kidneys are examined by bimanual palpation. The left hand is placed behind each lumbar region in turn, either across the bed for the left side or leaning over the patient and placing the left hand behind the left flank. The right hand is placed anteriorly and the patient asked to take a deep breath; the kidney can be felt moving in a cranial–caudal direction between the two hands.

3 Percussion

The value of percussion in identifying tenderness has been already mentioned. It is also valuable in looking for the edge of the liver and spleen, an enlarged bladder and fluid in the flank; the patient is then asked to roll in each direction to see if this fluid level moves (shifting dullness).

Examination is completed by exposing the groins, to look for inguinal and femoral herniae (page 15). In clinical practice, rectal examination is essential to find pelvic lesions. Although this is not expected in the qualifying examination, it is important to tell the examiner that you would usually undertake this procedure. After abdominal examination it is essential to reposition the patient and ensure they are well covered and comfortable.

Abdominal pain

Abdominal pain may be acute or chronic and in the acute case, the severity of the pain and the accompanying peritonism are important factors in determining the need for urgent surgical or other intervention. Such emergencies require nil by mouth with passage of a nasogastric tube if there is nausea or distention, and intravenous fluids if there is dehydration. The position and type of pain and accompanying jaundice, vomiting, dysphagia, diarrhoea, constipation and abdominal distention all help in the differential diagnoses, and direct a clinical examination and subsequent investigations.

Clinical examination includes general features starting with the hands for pulse rate, volume and dryness, and laxity of the dorsal skin to identify dehydration. Pallor and deformity of nails are found in anaemia, and palmar flush and Dupuytren's, and telangectasia in liver disease.

Specific examinations of the head and neck are of the conjunctiva over the sclera, for jaundice, and under the lower lid for the pallor of anaemia, and palpation of the root of the neck for malignant nodes.

Abdominal examination must be accompanied by appropriate exposure including of the groin to identify inguinal and femoral hernia carried out without embarrassment to patient or attendees.

Examination follows the usual inspection, palpation, percussion, auscultation, but, in severe tenderness, percussion rebound is a key manoeuvre to identify maximum points of tenderness; severe tenderness prevents even superficial palpation particularly in children. Painless gentle percussion also rules out any severe tenderness in unsuspecting malingerers, who over-react to palpation, making interpretation difficult.

STATION 1.1 *(Answers – page 167)*

History

A 24-year-old man presents to the Emergency Department with a history of bloody diarrhoea. You are the student on call with the medical team. Please take a history of the presenting complaint with a view to making a diagnosis.

(5 minute station)

STATION 1.2

History

You are a GP, new to this practice. Your next patient is a 42-year-old woman who has just returned from a foreign holiday with a 10-day history of diarrhoea. Please take a history of the presenting complaint, explaining to the patient the likely diagnosis and the investigations you wish carry out.

(10 minute station)

STATION 1.3

History

You are the medical student attached to a gastroenterology firm. You have been asked to take a history from a 24-year-old woman, who has been referred to the outpatient department by her GP with a 3- to 4-month history of 'diarrhoea'. Please take a history of her presenting complaint with a view to making a diagnosis. (You should be able to give a differential diagnosis at the end of the station.)

(5 minute station)

STATION 1.4

History

You are the medical student attached to the general medical firm on call. You have been asked by the registrar to clerk a 36-year-old woman who has just arrived in the Emergency Department after vomiting some blood. She is haemodynamically stable. Please take a history of the presenting complaint and any other relevant history with a view to making a diagnosis.

(5 minute station)

STATION 1.5

History

You are the medical student attached to a gastroenterology firm. You have been asked to take a history from a patient who has been referred to the outpatient department with epigastric pain and a proven microcytic anaemia. Please take a history of the presenting complaint and any other relevant history with a view to making a diagnosis.

(5 minute station)

STATION 1.6

History

Please answer the following questions, which are associated with the history you have just taken from the stockbroker in Station 1.5, indicating whether the statements are **True** or **False**.

(10 minute station)

	True	False
1 This patient should have an oesophago-gastroduodenoscopy	☐	☐
2 This patient will have a high plasma ferritin	☐	☐
3 This patient may have koilonychia	☐	☐
4 This patient will have a raised MCV	☐	☐
5 This patient should have a CLO test	☐	☐
6 This patient may require triple therapy	☐	☐
7 Triple therapy is given for 3 to 4 weeks	☐	☐
8 Clarithromycin is commonly used in triple therapy	☐	☐
9 Cimetidine is a proton pump inhibitor used in triple therapy	☐	☐
10 This patient will need to be on routine omeprazole for life	☐	☐

STATION 1.7

History

You are a GP. The next patient is a 47-year-old man who has come to see you with 'swallowing problems'. Please take a history of the presenting complaint and any other relevant history with a view to making a diagnosis.

(10 minute station)

STATION 1.8

History

You are the medical student attached to the medical team on call. You have been asked by the registrar to take a history from a 33-year-old man who has presented in the Emergency Department with jaundice. Please take a history of the presenting complaint and any other relevant history with a view to making a diagnosis.

(10 minute station)

STATION 1.9

History

You are a medical student attached to a surgical firm. A 65-year-old woman is referred to the surgical clinic by her GP complaining of abdominal symptoms and an alteration in her bowel habit. The consultant has asked you to take a history from this patient.

(5 minute station)

STATION 1.10

History

A 53-year-old man was referred to the surgical clinic complaining of intermittent bleeding per rectum and a fleshy lesion protruding through the anus. You are a medical student and the registrar has asked you to take a history from this patient.

(5 minute station)

STATION 1.11

Examination

You are a medical student on a gastroenterology firm. You have been asked by the SpR to examine this patient's abdomen. Please make a full assessment starting at the hands.

(10 minute station)

STATION 1.12

Examination

You are a medical student attached to a surgical firm. The SpR has asked you to examine this patient's abdomen. You should start at the abdomen ie you DO NOT need to examine the hands/face/chest. You may be asked questions at the end of this case.

(10 minute station)

STATION 1.13

Examination

You are a PRHO attached to a general medical firm. The next patient presented with jaundice five days ago which has subsequently resolved. Please make a full appropriate assessment to determine the possible causes.

(10 minute station)

STATION 1.14

Examination

You are a medical student attached to a surgical firm. This 8-year-old girl has presented with right iliac fossa pain which initially started periumbilically. Please make an appropriate abdominal assessment – starting at the hands. You will be asked some questions about the diagnosis and further management on completing your examination.

(10 minute station)

STATION 1.15

Examination

A 60-year-old man is admitted as an emergency to the surgical ward with a seven day history of increasingly severe cramp like abdominal pains in the left lower abdomen associated with nausea and constipation.

Please examine his abdomen with a view to making a diagnosis. You do not need to make a general examination of the patient but should make an assessment of his 'wellbeing'.

(10 minute station)

STATION 1.16

Examination

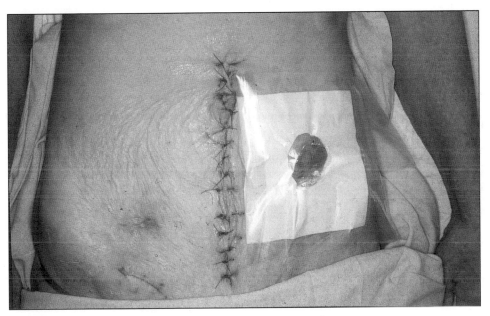

fig 1.16

Please examine this patient's abdomen (fig 1.16); describe your actions as you proceed and comment on your findings.

(5 minute station)

STATION 1.17

Examination

You are a medical student in the surgical outpatient department. The next patient is a fit and well 55-year-old man who presented with a longstanding lump in his right groin. This comes and goes but became tender and persistent for a few hours last week. Please examine this patient's lump (he is sitting in his underclothes on the side of the bed).

(5 minute station)

STATION 1.18

Examination

figs 1.18a, 1.18b, 1.18c and 1.18d show abnormalities of the tongue. Please make a diagnosis for each, and match one or more of the following statements to the illustrations.

(5 minute station)

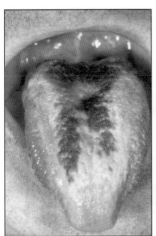

fig 1.18a

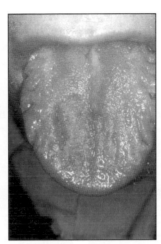

fig 1.18b

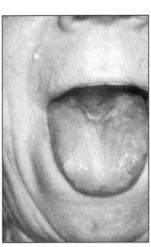

fig 1.18c

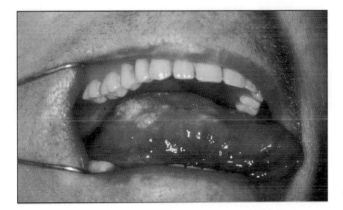

fig 1.18d

Statements	Figure
1 Is frequently a congenital condition	
2 Is usually asymptomatic	
3 Is caused by overgrowth of filiform papillae	
4 Is associated with tobacco smoking or chewing	
5 Is a pre-cancerous condition	
6 Is managed by regular oral hygiene	

STATION 1.19

Examination

Figs 1.19a and 1.19b are endoscopic views of the distal oesophagus and the gastric antrum respectively.

(5 minute station)

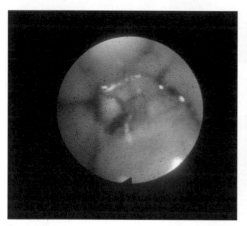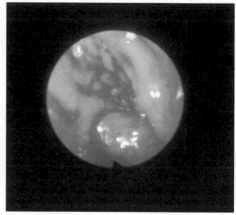

fig 1.19b   fig 1.19a

1 Please list the features observed in each
2 (a) State the probable diagnosis in each
    (b) How would you confirm your diagnosis in fig 1.19b?
3 State an aetiological factor associated with each of these conditions
4 List two symptoms in each that could lead a patient to seek medical advice

STATION 1.20

Examination

Figs 1.20a and 1.20b are colonoscopic findings in the transverse colon and rectum respectively.

(5 minute station)

1 Please list the features observed in each

2 What is the probable diagnosis in each?

3 (a) State the predisposing factor in fig 1.20a where the patient had been on long-term antibiotic therapy

   (b) State the probable sequelae of leaving the patient of fig 1.20b untreated

4 How would you treat both conditions?

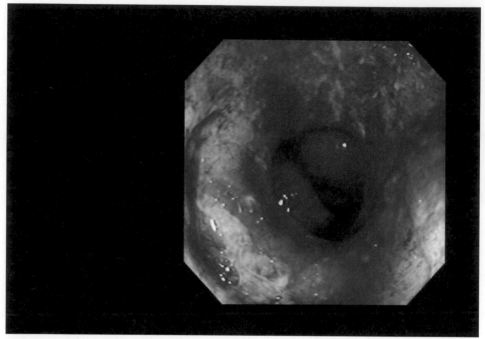

fig 1.20a

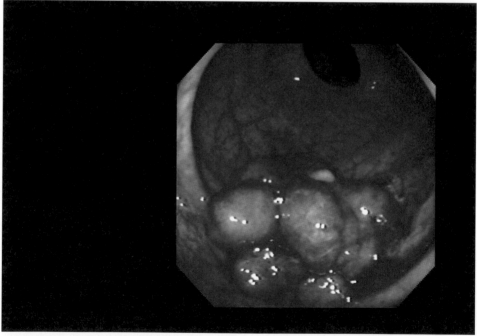

fig 1.20b

STATION 1.21

Investigation

The following patients are all attending the gastroenterology clinic. Please match the patient histories with the most appropriate diagnosis and full blood count result.

(5 minute station)

Patient history	Full blood count	Diagnosis
1 A 23-year-old woman with weight loss, lethargy and steatorrhoea	(A) Hb 9.9 MCV 67 WCC 10.3 Plats 302	(a) Peptic ulcer with disease
2 A 32-year-old with chronic liver disease and a raised red cell transketolase	(B) Hb 8.9 MCV 85 WCC 6.5 Plats 221	(b) Pernicious anaemia
3 A 54-year-old man with weight loss and constipation	(C) Hb 11.2 MCV 70 WCC 11.8 Plats 654	(c) Inflammatory bowel disease
4 A 74-year-old woman with known hyperthyroidism and a history of collapse	(D) Hb 7.5 MCV 104 WCC 3.9 Plats 64	(d) Coeliac disease
5 A 27-year-old man with epigastric pain and melaena	(E) Hb 9.2 MCV 105 WCC 4.7 Plats 353	(e) Alcoholic liver disease
6 A 29-year-old man with a two-year history of treated episodic bloody diarrhoea and mucous PR	(F) Hb 3.6 MCV 122 WCC 2.1 Plats 3.2	(f) Colonic carcinoma

Answers

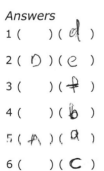

1 (   ) (d)

2 (D) (e)

3 (   ) (f)

4 (   ) (b)

5 (A) (a)

6 (   ) (C)

STATION 1.22

Investigation

The patients below have all presented with weight loss. Please match the patient histories with the most appropriate investigation results and diagnosis.

(5 minute station)

Patient history	Investigations	Diagnosis
1 A 67-year-old man with jaundice, pale stools and anorexia	(A) Albumin 23 Alk phos 232 AST 31 Bili 13 1.80 CCa^{2+} Amylase 23	(a) Colonic carcinoma with multiple metastases
2 A 52-year-old woman with palmar erythema, spider naevi and hepatosplenomegaly	(B) Albumin 24 Alk phos 454 AST 54 Bili 32 2.42 CCa^{++} Amylase 43	(b) Coeliac disease
3 A 25-year-old woman with steatorrhoea and general malaise	(C) Albumin 35 Alk phos 321 AST 93 Bili 124 1.92 CCa^{2+} Amylase 1098	(c) Carcinoma of the head of the pancreas
4 A 59-year-old man with weight loss, constipation and blood PR	(D) Albumin 26 Alk phos 607 AST 109 Bili 45 3.05 CCa^{2+} Amylase 32	(d) Acute pancreatitis
5 A 43-year-old obese woman with generalised abdominal pain and fever	(E) Albumin 21 Alk phos 644 AST 245 Bili 308 2.56 CCa^{2+} Amylase 204	(e) Primary biliary cirrhosis

Answers

1 (   ) (   )   4 (   ) (   )

2 (   ) (   )   5 (   ) (   )

3 (   ) (   )

STATION 1.23

Investigation

The following patients have presented to the hepatology clinic with deranged LFTs. Please match the patient histories with the most appropriate diagnosis and disease marker.

(5 minute station)

Patient history	Diagnosis	Marker
1 A 47-year-old man who has known chronic hepatitis B disease now presenting with hepatomegaly and weight loss	(A) Wilson's disease *E*	(a) Raised serum ferritin
2 A 58-year-old woman with recent weight loss and constipation	(B) Primary biliary cirrhosis *B*	(b) Antismooth muscle antibody
3 A 34-year-old man with diabetes, a 'suntan' and jaundice	(C) Colonic carcinoma *F* with metastases	(c) Antimitochondrial antibody
4 A 56-year-old woman with signs of chronic liver disease and periorbital xanthelasma	(D) Hepatoma *A*	(d) Low serum copper and caeruloplasmin
5 A 33-year-old woman with signs of chronic liver disease, jaundice and a cushingoid appearance	(E) Haemachromatosis *D*	(e) Alpha fetoprotein
6 A 39-year-old man with tremor, gait problems and Kaiser–Fleischer rings	(F) Autoimmune hepatitis *C*	(f) Markedly raised carcinoembryonic antigen

Answers

1 (D) (e)   4 (F) (b)

2 (C) (F)   5 (B) (C)

3 (E) (a)   6 (A) (d)

STATION 1.24

Investigation

Please indicate which of the statements regarding the patients a to d are **True** or **False**.

(5 minute station)

Patient	HBs Ag	aHBs Ig	HBc Ag	aHBc IgG IgM	HBe Ag	aHBe Ig
(a)	+	–	–	– +	+	–
(b)	–	+	–	– –	–	–
(c)	+	–	–	+ –	+	–
(d)	+	–	–	+ –	–	+

	True	False
1 Patient (a) has developed immunity to the hepatitis B virus	☐	☐
2 Patient (a) has evidence of acute viral replication	☐	☐
3 Patient (a) is a chronic carrier	☐	☐
4 Patient (b) has chronic active hepatitis	☐	☐
5 Patient (b) is immune to further infection with hepatitis B	☐	☐
6 Patient (b) is more susceptible to hepatoma	☐	☐
7 Patient (c) shows evidence of high-risk infectivity	☐	☐
8 Patient (c) may transmit the virus transplacentally	☐	☐
9 Patient (c) is at risk of cirrhosis	☐	☐
10 Patient (d) has chronic active hepatitis	☐	☐
11 Patient (d) shows evidence of low-risk infectivity	☐	☐
12 Patient (d) may still donate blood	☐	☐

STATION 1.25

Investigation

The following patients have all presented to their GP with diarrhoea. Please match the patient histories with the most appropriate causative organism and description.

(5 minute station)

Patient History	Organism	Description
1 A 73-year-old woman who ate luncheon meat at her club 24 hours ago. She now has profuse vomiting and diarrhoea and is hypotensive. Several other diners have been admitted to hospital	(A) *Clostridium difficile*	(a) Coccidian oocysts in faeces
2 A 22-year-old man who presents 24 hours after eating a reheated, luke-warm Chinese take away	(B) *Entamoeba histolytica*	(b) Flagellate protozoan
3 A 61-year-old man who has been on oral cefuroxime for ten days for a UTI	(C) *Cryptospiridiuim*	(c) Motile trophozoite
4 A 31-year-old man who has just returned from Russia with a five-day history of watery diarrhoea	(D) *Bacillus cereus*	(d) Gram negative lactose-fermenting rod
5 A 27-year-old woman who is HIV positive presenting with two weeks of profuse watery diarrhoea	(E) *Eschericia coli*	(e) Gram positive spore forming aerobic
6 A 32-year-old woman returns to England after teaching for a year in South East Asia. She is feeling listless and tired, with a six-week history of episodic watery diarrhoea, containing flecks of blood and mucus	(F) *Giardia lamblia*	(f) gram positive anaerobic

Answers

1 (   ) (   )

2 (   ) (   )

3 (   ) (   )

4 (   ) (   )

5 (   ) (   )

6 (   ) (   )

STATION 1.26

Investigation

The plain abdominal radiographs (figs 1.26a and 1.26b) are those of a 47-year-old man with a six-day history of colicky abdominal pain and vomiting.

(5 minute station)

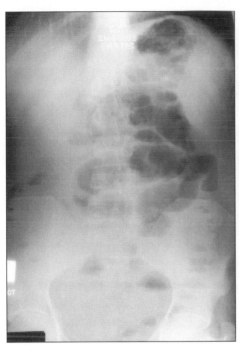
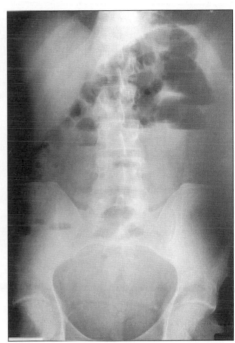

fig 1.26a   fig 1.26b

1 How were these two radiographs taken?

2 List the salient features of each

3 State your radiological diagnosis

4 List your definitive management

STATION 1.27

Investigation

A 33-year-old man suffering from AIDS developed abdominal cramps and constipation over two weeks. The result of a radiological investigation is shown in fig 1.27.

(5 minute station)

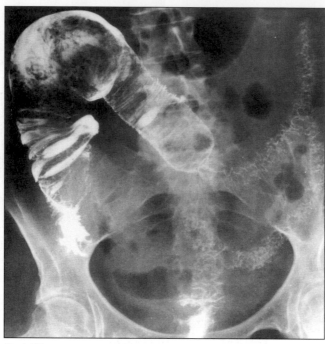

fig 1.27

1 Please name the investigation performed

2 How would you perform this investigation?

3 State the positive findings and your diagnosis

4 How would you treat this condition?

STATION 1.28

Investigation

The radiographs below are taken from patients presenting with abdominal pain.
Please indicate whether the statements are **True** or **False**.

(5 minute station)

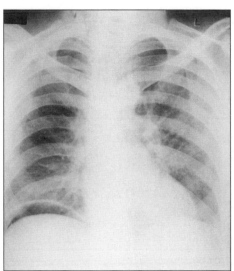

fig 1.28a

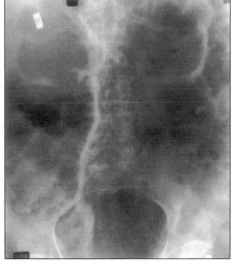

fig 1.28b

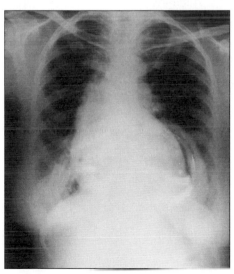

fig 1.28c

1 (fig 1.28a)	True	False
(a) This is an erect CXR	☐	☐
(b) The appearances are normal post-ERCP	☐	☐
(c) The appearances are normal two days post-laparoscopy	☐	☐
(d) There is evidence of a perforated viscus	☐	☐
(e) The patient should be treated initially by 'drip and suck'	☐	☐

2 (fig 1.28b)	True	False
(a) This is a supine AXR	☐	☐
(b) There is evidence of small bowel obstruction	☐	☐
(c) There are multiple fluid levels	☐	☐
(d) The caecum is loaded with faecal residue	☐	☐
(e) A common cause of this appearance is adhesions	☐	☐

2 (fig 1.28b)	True	False
(a) There is evidence of cardiomegaly	☐	☐
(b) There is evidence of free air in the peritoneum	☐	☐
(c) The LFTs will be normal in this case	☐	☐
(d) There may be a microcytosis on the blood film	☐	☐
(e) The features are consistent with gallstone ileus	☐	☐

STATION 1.29

Investigation

The patients below have all presented with dysphagia. Please indicate whether the statements are **True** or **False**.

(5 minute station)

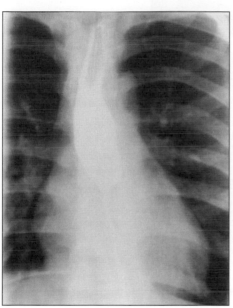

fig 1.29a

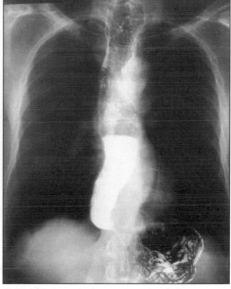

fig 1.29b

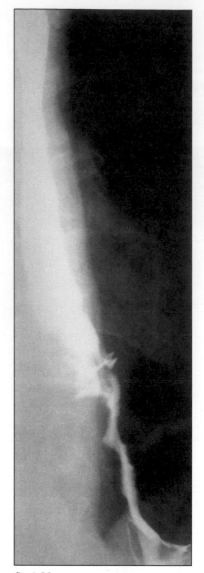

fig 1.29c

1 (fig 1.29a)	True	False
(a) This is a barium meal	☐	☐
(b) It shows a benign oesophageal stricture	☐	☐
(c) There is evidence of presbyoesophagus	☐	☐
(d) Impact pain is a common presenting symptom	☐	☐
(e) A common cause of this appearance is reflux oesophagitis	☐	☐

2 (fig 1.29b)	True	False
(a) This is a single contrast barium study	☐	☐
(b) The oesophageal lumen is within normal limits	☐	☐
(c) The appearances are caused by Barrett's oesophagus	☐	☐
(d) The condition shown is linked to cigarette smoking	☐	☐
(e) Patients are at increased risk of adenocarcinoma of the oesophagus	☐	☐

3 (fig 1.29c)	True	False
(a) This is a barium follow through study	☐	☐
(b) It shows severe peptic ulceration	☐	☐
(c) The disorder shown is common in Iran	☐	☐
(d) The condition may be cured by bismuth colloid	☐	☐
(e) YAG laser can be used to treat this condition	☐	☐

STATION 1.30

Investigation

The patients below have all presented with a microcytic anaemia and weight loss.
Please indicate whether the statements are **True** or **False**.

(5 minute station)

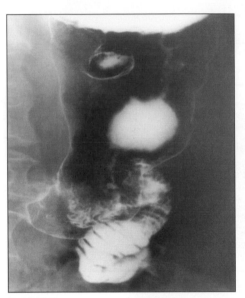

fig 1.30a

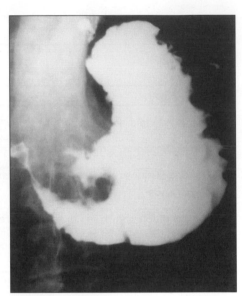

fig 1.30b

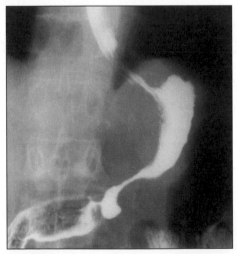

fig 1.30c

1 (fig 1.30a)	True	False
(a) This is a barium meal and follow through study	☐	☐
(b) There is evidence of gastric atrophy	☐	☐
(c) There is a benign ulcer in the pylorus of the stomach	☐	☐
(d) There are numerous jejunal and duodenal diverticulae	☐	☐
(e) This disorder is associated with *Campylobacter jejuni*	☐	☐

2 (fig 1.30b)	True	False
(a) This is a barium follow through study	☐	☐
(b) There is evidence of pyloric stenosis	☐	☐
(c) There is a large ulcer on the lesser curvature	☐	☐
(d) The disorder shown may be cured by triple therapy	☐	☐
(e) The disorder shown is associated with pernicious anaemia	☐	☐

3 (fig 1.30c)	True	False
(a) This is a barium meal and follow through study	☐	☐
(b) There is evidence of a duodenal ulceration	☐	☐
(c) The oesophagus is normal	☐	☐
(d) The stomach is abnormal	☐	☐
(e) The condition shown is referred to as linitis plastica	☐	☐

STATION 1.31

Investigation

The patients below have all presented with bleeding per rectum. Please indicate whether the statements are **True** or **False**

(5 minute station)

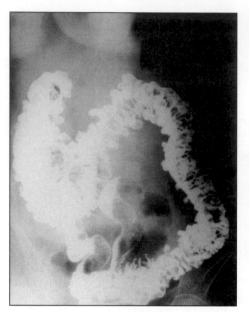

fig 1.31a

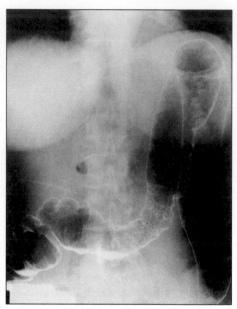

fig 1.31b

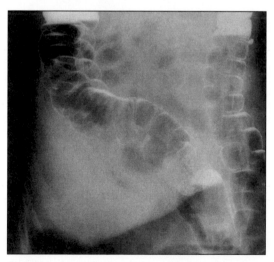

fig 1.31c

1 (fig 1.31a)	True	False
(a) This is a barium enema	☐	☐
(b) There has been poor bowel preparation	☐	☐
(c) This is a decubitus view	☐	☐
(d) The disorder shown is more common in black Africans	☐	☐
(e) This disorder is a complication of inflammatory bowel disease	☐	☐

1 (fig 1.31b)	True	False
(a) This is a single contrast barium study	☐	☐
(b) The loss of haustral pattern in the descending colon is termed 'lead piping'	☐	☐
(c) There is evidence of diverticulae	☐	☐
(d) The disorder shown is more common in women	☐	☐
(e) The patient is at increased risk of colonic carcinoma	☐	☐

1 (fig 1.31c)	True	False
(a) This is a double contrast study	☐	☐
(b) It shows a benign stricture of the transverse colon	☐	☐
(c) The stricture is sited in the distal transverse colon	☐	☐
(d) This stricture is almost certainly related to IBD	☐	☐
(e) This patient is probably in their 6th to 7th decade	☐	☐

STATION 1.32

Please label the CT scan of the abdomen shown below.

(5 minute station)

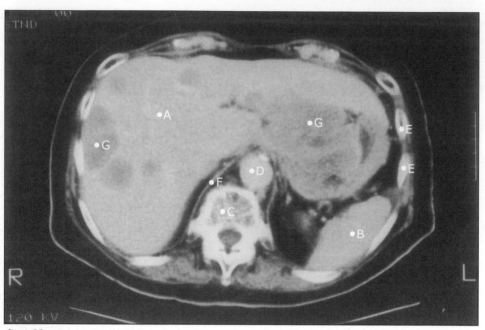

fig 1.32

Answers

(A)

(B)

(C)

(D)

(E)

(F)

(G)

STATION 1.33

Investigation

Please answer the questions regarding the investigations shown below.

(5 minute station)

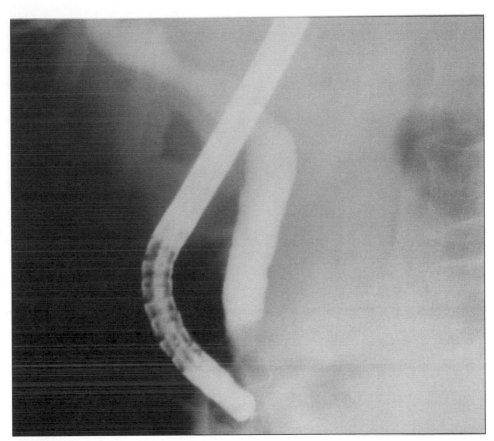

fig 1.33a

1 (fig 1.33a)

(a) What is this investigation?

(b) Describe the abnormalities

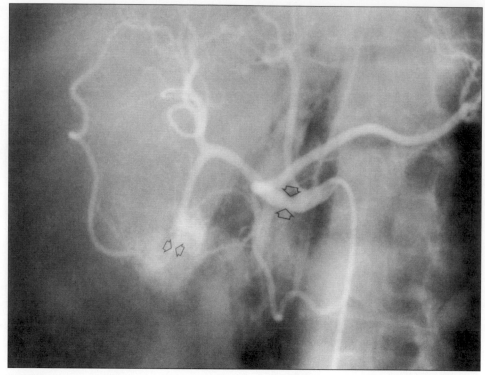

fig 1.33b

2 (fig 1.33b)

(a) What is this investigation?

(b) What are the structures labelled by the arrows?

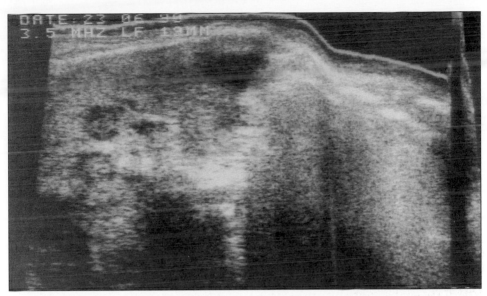

Fig. 1.33c

3 (fig 1.33c)

(a) What is this investigation?

(b) List three abdominal indications for it

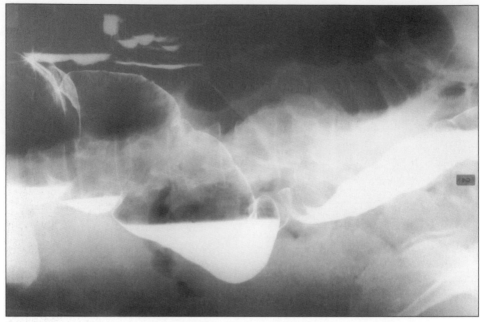

Fig. 1.33d

4 (fig 1.33d)

(a) What is this investigation?

(b) What is the major abnormality?

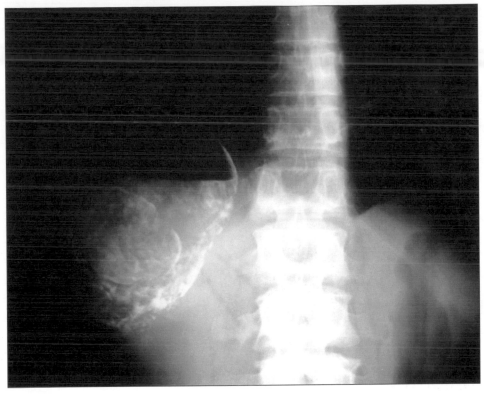

fig 1.33e

5 (fig 1.33e)

(a) What is this investigation?

(b) What is the major abnormality?

(c) List three differential causes

STATION 1.34

Therapueutics

A 23-year-old woman returns to outpatients for the results of her biopsies taken recently at OGD. The biopsy report is shown below.

'Areas of chronic inflammatory changes consistent with benign duodenal ulceration. *Helicobacter pylori* is also identified within this section.'

From the patient's details and drugs listed below please write out a prescription for this patient.

(5 minute station)

Mrs Helen Myers   Hospital Number 0136458   DOB 13/7/81
24 Gardenia Road
Cravenbrook
Middleton, M34 WNT

Drugs:

Ranitidine 300 mg nocte   Lansoprazole 30 mg bd
Metronidazole 400 mg bd   Clarithromycin 250 mg or 500 mg bd
Flucloxacillin 500 mg qds   Amoxycillin 750 mg tds or 1 g bd
Cimetidine 800 mg nocte   Omeprazole 20 mg bd
Misoprostol 400 mg bd   Tetracycline 250 mg qds
Ranitidine-bismuth citrate 400 mg bd

Hospital Number [ ] [ ] [ ] [ ] [ ] [ ]

Mr/Mrs/Ms Surname...

Forename...

Address ....

....

DOB   [ ] [ ] / [ ] [ ] / [ ] [ ]

Doctor's Signature..

Print Name...

Date   [ ] [ ] / [ ] [ ] / [ ] [ ]

STATION 1.35

Therapeutics

You are the house officer on a gastroenterology firm. You have been asked by the pharmacy to check a prescription for a TPN bag which has been ordered for one of your patients. The constituents of the bag and some of the patient's details are shown below.

(10 minute station)

Mr L B is a 27-year-old man who was admitted nine days ago after suffering a severe head injury in an RTA. He also suffered multiple fractures of the lower limbs. Since admission he has been electively paralysed and ventilated on the intensive care unit. He has had TPN running for three days and has a post-traumatic small gut ileus. Today he has a temperature of 38.5°C. He is at present haemodynamically stable.

He has a triple lumen central venous line in situ, an indwelling urinary catheter and a pelvic external fixator.

Height:1.80 m   Weight: 80 kg

His most recent investigations are:

FBC: Hb 10.5,   WCC 14.6,   platelets 355
U+Es: Na$^+$ 139, K$^+$ 2.6, bicarbonate 21, urea 21, creatinine 399
Glucose 17.5
Calcium 1.90, albumin 24, phosphate 1.0
Magnesium 0.61
CXR: Several rib fractures
CT head scan: generalised cerebral oedema and contusions

TPN constituents
Na$^+$ 80 mmol
K$^+$ 80 mmol
Protein 14 g
kcals 2650 – (fat 1000 kcals; carbohydrate 1300 kcals; protein 350 kcals)
Calcium 10 mmol
Phosphate 20 mmol
Magnesium 7.5 mmol
Volume 2.5 l

Please indicate whether the following statements are **True** or **False**.

	True	False
1 This patient is likely to be in an anabolic state	☐	☐
2 He has normal renal function	☐	☐
3 His corrected calcium is within normal limits	☐	☐
4 He does not require more than 40 mmol K$^+$ per day	☐	☐
5 He should have insulin added to his TPN bag	☐	☐
6 He should not have a high protein concentration in his TPN	☐	☐
7 His BMI is indicative of malnutrition	☐	☐
8 He can have all his fluid requirements given by TPN	☐	☐
9 Sepsis will not affect his TPN requirements	☐	☐
10 The TPN can be given through his central venous line	☐	☐

STATION 1.36

Procedures

The instruments (A) to (Γ) shown in fig 1.36 are all used in gastroenterological procedures. Please indicate whether the statements below are **True** or **False**.

(10 minute station)

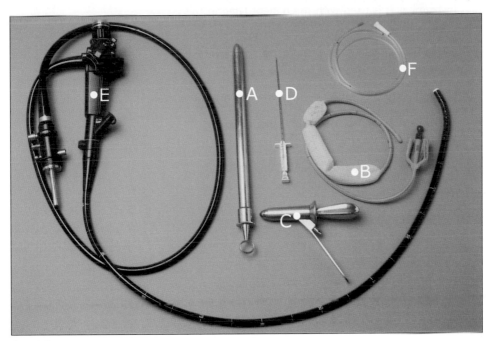

fig 1.36

	True	False
1 Instrument A is used to look directly into the oesophagus	☐	☐
2 Colonic biopsies may be taken through instrument A	☐	☐
3 Instrument A should only be inserted with local anaesthetic	☐	☐
4 Instrument B has become obselete because of the use of endoscopy	☐	☐
5 A tennis ball is often attached to one end of instrument B to stop the patient swallowing it	☐	☐
6 Instrument B is used to stop oesophagogastric variceal bleeding	☐	☐

	True	False
7 Instrument C is principally used to view the rectum	☐	☐
8 Instrument C should always be used before using instrument A	☐	☐
9 Instrument C is also used for vaginal examination		
10 Instrument D is used with the patient lying in the left lateral position	☐	☐
11 The patient should have a check FBC and clotting screen prior to the use of instrument D	☐	☐
12 Instrument D is only used with a general anaesthetic	☐	☐
13 Instrument E can not be used to diagnose coeliac disease	☐	☐
14 Instrument E can cause a pneumomediastinum	☐	☐
15 Instrument E is used in ERCP	☐	☐
16 One indication to use instrument F is in a patient with a stroke	☐	☐
17 Instrument F is radio-opaque	☐	☐
18 Instrument F may be used for parenteral feeding	☐	☐

Chapter 2:
Neurology and Psychiatry

Contents

Neurology History

Psychiatry History

Neurological Examination

Chapter 2

Neurology and Psychiatry

Neurology History

Headache
- **Site**
- **Radiation**
- **Character**
  Dull, severe, sharp
- **Duration and onset**
  Sudden: subarachnoid haemorrhage, meningitis, migraine
  Insidious: raised intracranial pressure, migraine
- **Exacerbating factors**
  Early morning or after periods of lying down
  Straining at stool
  Laughing
  Coughing: associated with raised intracranial pressure
- **Relieving factors**
  Analgesia: paracetamol, NSAIDs, opiates
- **Precipating factors**
  Stress
  Oral contraceptive pill (may precipitate several causes of headache including migraine, sagittal vein thrombosis and benign intracranial hypertension)
  Specific foods
  Alcohol
- **Associated factors**
  Nausea and vomiting, photophobia, neck stiffness
  Fever
  Rashes
  Pharyngitis, cough, sputum, myalgia, arthralgia
  Seizures
  Decreased level of consciousness/coma

Blackouts

May be caused by seizures, TIAs, strokes and decreased cerebral perfusion.

- **Seizures**
  Pre-warning aura
  Urinary incontinence
  Tongue biting
  Amnesia
  Facial appearance – cyanosed or pale
  Tonic–clonic episodes
  Head injury/trauma
  One should try to find witnesses to the 'fit' to corroborate the history
- **TIAs/stroke**
  Associated motor/sensory deficit
- **Vertebro-basilar insufficiency**
  Classically loss of consciousness associated with looking upwards and/or cervical spondylosis
- **Carotid hypersensitivity**
  Classically associated with tight collars and ties
- **Speech/comprehension problems**
- **Dysphasia**
  Receptive/expressive
- **Dysarthria**
  This may be associated with swallowing problems and nasal regurgitation of food

Visual disturbances

- **Amaurosis fugax**
  Sudden 'curtain of darkness' or black spots covering the visual field. It is associated with thromboembolic phenomenon: loss of visual fields, eg tunnel vision, bitemporal hemianopia, blurring/loss of vision, zig-zag lines preceding migraines

Motor/sensory deficit

Motor weakness may be described as global, hemiparesis, paraparesis, proximal or distal; lower motor neurone disorders are associated with wasting and fasciculation.

It is traditional, in cases of weakness to start a neurology clerking by mentioning the dominant hand of the patient, ie **This 34-year-old right-handed man**...

In patients presenting with weakness in the lower limbs it is important to exclude symptoms of cord compression. The weakness and associated symptoms are usually acute but may be insidious in onset.

Associated symptoms include:

- **Paraparesis**
  Weakness of the lower limbs
- **Sensory loss**
  A sensory level should be defined:
  - T4 – nipple
  - T10 – umbilicus
  - T12 – above the inguinal ligament
  - L1 – below the inguinal ligament
- Constipation
- Urinary retention

Sensory changes include parasthesiae and numbness. Peripheral sensory neuropathy classically occurs in a 'glove and stocking' distribution.

Dizziness

Associated with vestibular, brainstem and cerebellar disorders. It is important to determine associated hearing loss, tinnitus and vomiting.

Psychiatry History

The history in psychiatry plays an important part in making the correct diagnosis. It is important to ask broad, open questions within the framework of a specific history. The OSCE format can be limiting in this respect, as time constraints may force a more concise, directed approach. However, the student must try to bring into the histories a sense of empathy associated with this directioned approach, without losing sight of making a diagnosis.

Presenting complaint: psychosis versus neurosis

This is the principal differentiating factor between psychosis and neurosis. Neurotics rarely lose sight of reality and normally have good insight into their illness and problems.

First rank symptoms
Psychotic symptoms displayed by schizophrenics

- Auditory hallucination
- Thought withdrawal and insertion
- Thought broadcasting
- Delusional perception
- Somatic passivity
- External control of emotions

The differential diagnosis of acute psychosis includes recreational drug abuse, which must be excluded in the history.

Depression
- Low mood
- Depressed view of present and future
- Early morning wakening, poor/disturbed sleep patterns
- Poor appetite
- Loss of enthusiasm
- Lack of self-interest and interest in the environment

Self-harm/suicidal thoughts
All patients should be asked about suicidal thoughts and ideation (ie formulation of suicide attempt).

Mania
Elevated mood, increased energy, decreased sleep, grandiose ideas; delusions of grandeur, forced speech, flight of ideas, increased libido.

Suicidal intent
It is extremely important to be able to make an accurate assessment of suicidal intent. The consequences of an incorrect assessment can be fatal. All patients presenting with deliberate self-harm should have a formal psychiatric assessment prior to discharge from hospital. Important factors include:

- Age – deliberate self-harm is rarely just a cry for help in the elderly. They are, therefore, often successful in attempts to commit suicide and rarely present to hospital
- Planning
- Method
- Suicide note and content
- Premorbid events – precipitating factors, (eg loss of job, marital split, bereavement)
- Family/personal history of deliberate self-harm
- Family/personal history of psychiatric illness
- Present view of suicidal attempt
- View of the future
- Symptoms of depression

Drug and alcohol abuse
- Alcohol abuse – duration
  Units of alcohol per 24 hours (1 unit: 1 glass of wine, 1 measure of spirits, ½ pint of regular strength beer or lager)
  Always ask about all three types of alcohol – wine, beer and spirits
- View of alcohol excess – patients must see drinking as a problem and be prepared to accept help offered. Their view may be judged by the CAGE questionnaire
- Drinking patterns – drinking alone, in the mornings, to relieve symptoms of withdrawal
- Previous attempts at 'drying out'/withdrawal – formal and informal
- Previous admissions for delirium tremens, GI bleeds or pancreatitis

Recreational drug use
- Type – amphetamines, sedatives, cannabis, opiates
- Method – tablets, intravenous injection, smoking
- Duration of abuse
- View of drug taking
- Understanding of withdrawal
- Alcohol, cigarette smoking and illicit drug abuse are often associated and one should always ask about the others when taking a history

Other important elements of the psychiatric history
- Premorbid personality
- Perceptions of their present illness
- View of the future
- Family history – particularly psychiatric illness
- Previous medical and psychiatric history
- Medications
- Childhood, schooling, further education
- Occupational history
- Criminal history
- Sexual history (may be relevant in certain cases)
- Major life events – bereavement, economic hardship, unemployment, divorce

Neurological Examination

Neurological assessment is often the medical student's nemesis. It requires a lot of practice and reading around the subject. It truly is the 'appliance of science'!

Cranial nervous system

To assess the cranial nervous system within the limitations of OSCEs and traditional short cases they are often grouped into their anatomical divisions.

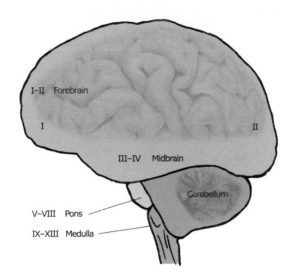

Stations are thus divided into:

1 Examination of the eyes and extra-ocular muscles. Cranial nerves II, III, IV and VI
2 Examination of cranial nerves V, VII, VIII (pontine)
3 Examination of cranial nerves IX, X, XI, XII (medulla or bulbar nerves)

1 Examination of the eyes and extra-ocular muscles. Cranial nerves II, III, IV and VI
(Note – Ophthalmoscopy is covered in chapter 3 (see diabetic retinopathy).)

Introduce yourself with name and role; explain the examination and gain verbal consent to proceed.

Observation – look for signs of asymmetry between the two eyes: ptosis, constriction or dilatation of pupils, exophthalmos and general signs of stroke disease eg hemiparesis and other cranial nerve lesions eg facial palsy.

OSCE Stations

Visual acuity – ask the patient 'Do you normally wear glasses?' If so assess the eyes with the glasses on and off. Always examine one eye then the other. Test BEST acuity through the following tests:

- Reading text: if available use a Snellen chart at 6 m and ask the patient 'please read the lowest/smallest line that you can'. Otherwise use newspaper print or other easily available reading material
- Counting fingers: if the patient is unable to read the largest print ask them to count fingers at 1 m
- Perception of movement: if unable to see fingers ask them 'Tell me when you see my fingers wiggle/move'
- Perception of light: turn a pen torch on and off and ask the patient to tell you when they can see the light
- Blindness – unable to perceive changes of light

Visual fields – check all four quadrants of each eye
Perform the test at 1 m apart comparing your fields (hopefully normal) with that of the patient.

- Ask the patient to cover the eye not being tested
- Close/cover your corresponding eye
- Hold up your index finger and gently wiggle it while keeping your upper limb fully extended and ask 'can you see the finger move?'

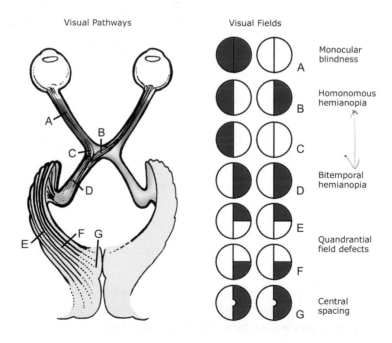

Visual Pathways   Visual Fields

A Monocular blindness

B Homonomous hemianopia

C

D Bitemporal hemianopia

E

F Quandrantial field defects

G Central spacing

If 'yes' – the patient has a clinically normal or 'full' quadrant. There is no need to then move your finger inwards to the centre of field. Repeat in each of the four quadrants.

If 'no' – slowly move your finger in towards the centre of the visual field. Ask the patient to tell you when they see the finger moving. Record the reduction in the field.

Common abnormalities

1 Bitemporal hemianopia
2 Homonymous hemianopia
3 Homonymous quadrantanopia
4 Unilateral hemi/quadrantonopia
5 Lesions anterior to chiasma produce unilateral eye/visual loss
6 Lesions at optic chiasma classically produce bitemporal hemianopia – but may produce many other bilateral changes
7 Lesions posterior to chiasma lead to bilateral homonymous visual loss within the contralateral visual field, ie right homonymous hemianopia, may be due to left cortical or optic tract lesions

Once you have examined for field defects you may also wish to test for visual inattention (this is perhaps more relevant in clinical practice). Performing the test at 1 m apart, ask the patient to look directly into your eyes. In sequence wiggle your outstretched right index finger, the patient should point to the finger that is moving, then wiggle the left index finger, the patient will again point to the moving finger. However when both fingers are moved at the same time, the patient will only point to one of the fingers, indicating inattention to the opposite side.

Extra-ocular muscles (EOM)
Cranial nerve III (oculomotor n.) supplies all the EOM except:

IV (Trochlear n.) – superior oblique muscle
VI (Abducent n.) lateral rectus muscle (LR_6 SO_4)

Test the muscles in each direction of gaze. You should trace out an 'H'. Ask 'tell me if you see double at any point'. You should also specifically check for nystagmus.

Pupillary size, shape and symmetry; pupillary responses/reflexes

Check:

- Size and shape
- Symmetry
- Reaction to light – direct and consensual reaction – shining the light in one eye produces a direct response in that eye and a consensual (similar) response in the opposite eye.
- Accommodation

Once you have completed acuity, fields EOMs, pupillary responses, then offer to perform ophthalmoscopy.

2 Examination of the cranial nerves V, VII and VIII (pontine)
Trigeminal nerve, V

Motor: V supplies the muscles of mastication. Ask the patient to:

- Bite down/clench their teeth – palpate temporalis, masseters and pterygoids
- Open mouth – move jaw left and right. If there is weakness of motor function on one side the mandible will move TOWARDS the lesion, being pushed across by the normal pterygoids on the opposite side

Sensory: test light touch and/or pin prick in the three divisions of the V nerve (ophthalmic, mandibular and maxillary); compare one side with the other, right and left.

Corneal reflex – You should know how to perform the corneal reflex (although this is rarely performed in exam situations, candidates may be asked to explain how to do the procedure).

Facial nerve, VII

Motor supply to facial muscles
UMN lesion – sparing of the forehead
LMN lesion – complete hemifacial palsy

Ask the patient to:

- Smile/show their teeth – observe for asymmetry
- Blow out their cheeks – palpate for weakness
- Screw up their eyes – gently try to pull eye lids apart
- Look up to the ceiling – observe for asymmetry and loss of 'brow' markings

The VII nerve is also the sensory supply to the anterior two-thirds of the tongue.

Vestibulocochlear nerve, VII

Informally one can test hearing by covering one of the patient's ears and whispering into the other, asking the patient to repeat the whispered phrase back to you.

Carry out:

- Weber's test – if positive ie lateralises to one side, this simply demonstrates 'there is a problem'
- Rinne's test – confirms which side the problem is actually on. A normal response is considered a POSITIVE test and occurs when air conduction is better that bone conduction (AC>>BC [remembered A–B–C]), a NEGATIVE test is where bone conduction is better than air (BC>AC)

3 Examination of the cranial nerves IX, X, XI, XII (medulla or bulbar nerve)
Glossopharyngeal and vagus nerves, IX/X

Previously a candidate would be expected to test the 'gag' reflex. Today one would test.

- **Palatal sounds** 'say EGG or RUG', 'K or G' observe palatal movements. Note the palate moves AWAY from the side of lesion
- **Swallow**

To assess a patient's swallow they must be:

- Fully conscious ie not drowsy
- Able to follow commands
- Sitting upright, ie not lying flat

Ask patient to:

- Take a sip of water saying 'don't swallow it yet'
- 'Now swallow it' – observe for initiation of swallowing mechanism
- 'Now say your name' – listen for 'wet' voice indicating orophanyngeal pooling
- Throughout observe for coughing or choking.

Accessory nerve, XI

Motor supply
- Sternomastoids:
  - place one hand on the patient's forehead asking patient to push head up, off the pillow
  - observe and palpate for bulk and power of sternomastoids
- Trapezius – ask patient to shrug shoulders. Observe for asymmetry. If not obvious try to overcome shoulder shrug

Hypoglossal nerve, XII

Tongue: ask the patient to 'open mouth'. Observe tongue for wasting and fasciculation. 'Now please stick your tongue out' – watch for abnormal deviation. The tongue moves towards the side of the lesion.

Cerebellar assessment

Cerebellar signs are ipsilateral to lesions. Bilateral signs are normally termed a cerebellar syndrome.

Signs of cerebellar dysfunction are:

Dysdiadokokinesia
Ataxia
Nystagmus
Intention tremor
Slurred/staccato speech
Hypotonia/reflexia

However, this is not a helpful acronym for examination.The examination starts at the hands. Thus it becomes:

1 HANDS – dysdiadochokinesia and intention tremor
2 UPPER LIMBS – hypotonia/reflexia
3 EYES – nystagmus
4 Slurred/staccato speech
5 Ataxia truncal and gait

Common causes of unilateral lesions:

- Stroke – haemorrhage and infarct
- Space-occupying lesions:
    - benign (abscess)
    - malignant primaries – rare, secondaries – breast
- Demyelination

Cerebellar syndromes – (bilateral/global cerebellar dysfunction)

- Any of the causes of unilateral disease affecting both cerebellar lobes, ie stroke, space-occupying lesions and demyelination
- Toxins – principally alcohol
- Drugs – antiepileptics
- Paraneoplastic syndrome
- Congenital disorders (uncommon)
    - Dandy–Walker syndrome
    - Arnold–Chiari malformation

Peripheral nervous system (PNS)
Upper and lower limbs.

1 Motor examination

Patterns of weakness:
- Proximal vs distal eg proximal myopathy
- Upper motor neurone (UMN) vs lower motor neurone (LMN)
- In the distribution of peripheral nerves eg median nerve

Table 1

Upper motor neurone (UMN) vs lower motor neurone (LMN): this is the classical differentiation of a patient complaining of 'weakness'.

	UMN lesions	LMN lesions
Bulk	Normal	Wasting may be associated with fasciculation
Tone	Increased	Reduced
Power	Reduced	Reduced
Co-ordination	Note – if power is significantly reduced one cannot assess co-ordination in any meaningful manner	
Reflexes	Increased May be associated with clonus	Reduced or absent
Plantars	Extensor/upgoing	Flexor/downgoing
To summarise	Everything increases: • Tone • Reflexes • Upgoing (extensor) plantars	Everything decreases: • Tone • Reflexes • Downgoing (flexor) plantars

Grading of power

    0 – no movement

    1 – flicker of movement

    2 – movement but not against gravity

    3 – movement against gravity, easily overcome

    4 – movement against gravity but overcome

    5 – normal power

Grading of reflexes

    0 – absent

    1 – reduced

    2 – normal

    3 – increased (check for clonus)

When testing motor/sensory systems, always compare one side with the other. Eg shoulder abduction on right vs left or dermatomes of right with left.

UPPER LIMB

Assess bulk, tone, power, co-ordination, reflexes.

1 Bulk and tone

2 Power: ALWAYS COMPARE right versus left

- Shoulder abduction and adduction
- Elbow
  - o flexion (biceps)
  - o extension (triceps)
- Wrist – palmar and dorsiflexion
- Finger – abduction
- Thumb – abduction and opposition (both median nerve functions)

3 Reflexes

- Triceps jerk (root value C7, 8)
- Biceps jerk (C5, 6)
- Supinator jerk (C5, 6)

Lower limb

Assess bulk, tone, power, co-ordination, reflexes

1 Bulk and tone

2 Power: ALWAYS COMPARE right versus left

- Hip
  - flexion
  - extension
- Knee
  - flexion
  - extension
- Ankle
  - dorsiflexion
  - plantar flexion
- Foot
  - inversion
  - eversion

3 Reflexes

- Patella jerk (L3, 4)
- Ankle jerk (S1, 2)

Reflex	Root values of the reflexes '1 to 8'
Triceps jerk	(C) 7, 8
Biceps jerk	(C) 5, 6
Supinator jerk	(C) 5, 6
Patella jerk	(L) 3, 4
Ankle jerk	(S) 1, 2

The root values of the reflexes are as simple as remembering how to count from 1 to 8 (S1,2 – L3,4 – C5,6 – C5,6 – C7,8)

4 Gait – when asked to assess the motor system of the lower limbs you should ask to see the patient walk to assess their 'gait'. (see page 76)

(see page 76)

OSCE Stations

2 Sensory examination

To perform a competent sensory examination you will need to have an understanding of:

1   Patterns of sensory loss
- Dermatomal defining a 'sensory level' to localise a spinal lesion
- Peripheral sensory neuropathy: the classical 'glove and stocking' distribution
- Distribution of a peripheral nerve

2   Modalities to assess and their pathways
- Light touch, vibration, joint position or proprioception are carried by the dorsal columns
- Pain (pin prick), temperature carried by the spinothalamic tracts

3   Dermatomes – to make things easier to assess always place the patient in the 'anatomical position'

Dermatome representations vary between illustrations. The points shown on the diagrams below are invariably correct.

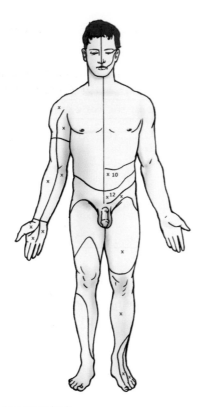

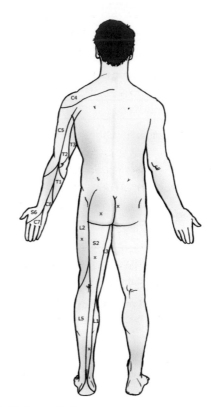

fig 2a Upper limb   fig 2b Lower limb

Conduct the following tests:

A light touch and pin prick

1 With patient's eyes open, test a normal area with pin (pain) or cotton wool (light touch). Ask 'does this feel sharp?' or 'does this feel soft?'

Note – a normal area of skin is taken as the skin overlying the sternal notch

2 Now explain – 'I'm going to move this down your arms/legs, tell me if it feels sharp/soft' – 'say yes if it feels sharp/soft' (the patient cannot say no if their eyes are truly shut!)
3 Then say 'now shut your eyes'
4 Compare one dermatome on the right with the corresponding one on the left
5 Move down the dermatomes – try to define sensory level or glove and stocking peripheral neuropathy

Vibration

1 Place a ringing tuning fork on the superior aspect of manubrium. Ask 'can you feel it buzzing/ringing?'
2 Explain 'I will place it on your hands/feet' – tell me if you feel it buzzing
3 Then say 'now shut your eyes.'

Place on bony prominences described below, left then right. You need only proceed to the next proximal point if the patient is unable to feel the ringing of the fork. Test the following areas:

- Upper limb
  - Interphalangeal joint of thumb
  - Metacarpophalangeal joint of thumb
  - Radial aspect of the wrist
  - Olecranon process at the elbow

- Lower limb
  - Interphalangeal joint of big toe
  - Metatarsophalangeal joint of big toe
  - Medial malleolus
  - Tibial tuberosity
  - Anterior superior iliac spine

Proprioception or joint position sense (JPS)

With the patient's eyes open:

1 Hold the tip of thumb or big toe with minimal contact
2 Move the tip 'up or down' a millimetre or two (only)
3 Ask 'can you tell the difference between up and down?' **If the patient can't tell the difference with their eyes open there is no point testing with eyes closed**!
4 'now close your eyes' – move the digit up or down asking them to tell you in which direction you are moving it

Test at levels:
- Interphalangeal joint
- metacarpo/tarsophalangeal joint
- wrist/ankle
- elbow/knee

Coordination

Coordination is part of the cerebellar assessment; thus, in the upper limb it is tested through dysdiadokinesia and past pointing and in the lower limbs through assessment of gait ataxia and the heel/shin test.

Heel/shin test

Ask the patient to lift their heel to their patella and then run it down the front of the shin to the ankle. LIFTING the foot up off the skin, replacing at the patella and repeat. A valid assessment of coordination can only be made if the patient has enough muscle power to sustain the required movement. Assessing the coordination of a patient with grade 3+/5 is therefore invalid.

Gait assessment

If you ask to see the patient walk you will need to know how to describe any abnormalities.

Classical gait abnormalities:

- Antalgic – due to pain/arthritis
- Parkinsonian – 'shuffling'
- Sensory ataxia – 'high-stepping/slapping'
- Cerebellar ataxia – wide-based/staggering gait
- Trendelenburg gait – due to OA/hip abnormalities

STATION 2.1 *(Answers – page 221)*

History

You are a medical student attending a neurology outpatient clinic. The first patient is a 21-year-old woman who has been referred by her GP with headaches. Please take a history of the presenting complaint and any other relevant history with a view to making a diagnosis.

(5 minute station)

STATION 2.2

History

You are a medical student attached to a GP practice. The next patient is a 19-year-old man with headaches. Please take a history of the presenting complaint and any other relevant history with a view to making a diagnosis.

(5 minute station)

STATION 2.3

History

You are a house officer attached to a busy medical firm. The registrar has asked you to take a history in the Emergency Department from a 23-year-old woman with a severe headache. Please take a history of the presenting complaint and any other relevant history with a view to making a diagnosis.

(5 minute station)

STATION 2.4

History

You are a medical student attending a neurology outpatient clinic. The next patient has been referred by his GP for 'funny turns'. Please take a history of the presenting complaint and any other relevant history with a view to making a diagnosis.

(5 minute station)

STATION 2.5

History

You are a house officer attached to a neurology firm. The next patient has been admitted from the consultant outpatient clinic for investigation of 'weakness'. Please take a history of the presenting complaint and any other relevant history with a view to making a diagnosis.

(5 minute station)

STATION 2.6

History

You are a medical student attached to a neurology firm. The next patient is a 62-year-old man who has been referred by his GP complaining of swallowing problems, weakness and weight loss. He is described as being very 'wasted'. Please take a history of the presenting complaint and any other relevant history with a view to making a diagnosis.

(5 minute station)

STATION 2.7

History

You are a house officer attached to a neurology firm. The next patient is a 24-year-old professional football player who has been referred by his GP with numbness and parasthesiae in the hands and feet associated with blurring of his vision. Please take a history of the presenting complaint and any other relevant history with a view to making a diagnosis. Following the consultation, name three investigations you would request for this patient.

(10 minute station)

STATION 2.8

History

You are a medical student attached to a GP practice. The next patient is a 54-year-old man who, while out shopping yesterday, had a strange turn where his left arm and leg went 'suddenly weak and dead' but recovered within 30 or 40 minutes. Please take a history of the presenting complaint and associated risk factors and counsel this man about lifestyle changes.

(10 minute station)

STATION 2.9

Examination

You are a medical student in the neurology outpatient clinic. The next patient has presented with weakness in the upper and lower limbs. Please perform a full motor examination – assessing the **upper** limbs only. **You do not need to assess the sensory system**.

(5 minute station)

STATION 2.10

Examination

You are a medical student in the neurology outpatient clinic. The next patient has presented with weakness in the upper and lower limbs. Please perform a full motor examination – assessing the **lower** limbs only. **You do not need to assess the sensory system**.

(5 minute station)

STATION 2.11

Examination

You are a medical student in medical outpatients. The next patient has presented with 'pins and needles' and numbness in his/her hands and feet. Please perform a sensory examination of their **upper limbs**.

(5 minute station)

STATION 2.12

Examination

You are a medical student in medical outpatients. The next patient has presented with 'pins and needles' and numbness in his/her hands and feet. Please perform a sensory examination of his/her **lower limbs**.

(5 minute station)

STATION 2.13

Examination

You are a medical student attached to a medical firm. The next patient was admitted in the early hours of the morning on the acute medical take having 'gone off their legs'. The patient has not passed any urine in 24 hours and is constipated. The patient has also had mid-lower thoracic back pain for the last 2–3 weeks. Please make a full neurological assessment (motor and sensory examinations) of the patient's lower limbs.

(10 minute station)

STATION 2.14

Examination

You are a medical student attached to a medical firm. The next patient was admitted from outpatients with 'cerebellar signs'. Please perform an appropriate examination to assess the patient for cerebellar signs.

(5 minute station)

STATION 2.15

Examination

You are a medical student attached to a neurology firm. The SpR has asked you to examine this patient's eyes with a view to making a diagnosis. Please perform a full examination of their eyes. You will be asked some questions at the end of your examination.

(10 minute station)

STATION 2.16

Examination

You are a medical student in medical outpatients. You have been asked by the SpR to assess this patient's visual fields. Please assess his/her fields with a view to making a diagnosis. You will be shown a diagram of the visual pathways to point out where you think the lesion may be.

(5 minute station)

STATION 2.17

Examination

You are a medical student attached to a medical firm. You have been asked by the consultant to examine this patient's cranial nerves, starting at cranial nerve V. Please make a full assessment of cranial nerves V to XII.

(10 minute station)

STATION 2.18

Examination

You are a medical student attached to a stroke unit. You have been asked by the nurse specialist to assess this patient's speech and swallow prior to him/her being referred to the speech and language therapist. You will need to decide whether they are safe to continue with oral intake or are to be made 'nil by mouth'.

(10 minute station)

STATION 2.19

Investigation

Each of the following patients had suffered an intracranial vascular event. Please match the haematological results with the patients' histories and diagnoses.

(5 minute station)

Patient history	Haematology result	Diagnosis
1 A 69-year-old man with severe chronic airways disease	(A) INR 2.8 Plats 22	(a) Drug-induced coagulopathy
2 A 37-year-old woman with spontaneous bruising, recurrent infection and intracerebral haemorrhage	(B) INR 9.4	(b) Autocoagulation, and thrombocytopenia
3 A 51-year-old woman with recent DVT and thrombosis of the right upper limb	(C) Hb 19.2 Hct 0.59	(c) Pancytopenia secondary to aplastic anaemia
4 A 41-year-old alcohol abuser	(D) Hb 11.4 WCC 5.9 Plats 2076	(d) Secondary polycythaemia
5 A 39-year-old woman with a prosthetic mitral valve, on erythromycin for chest infection now presenting in coma	(E) Hb 6.2 WCC 2.1 Plats 6	(e) Primary thrombocythaemia

Answers

1 (   ) (   )

2 (   ) (   )

3 (   ) (   )

4 (   ) (   )

5 (   ) (   )

STATION 2.20

Investigation

The following patients have presented with seizures. Please match the patient histories with the most likely biochemical abnormality and diagnosis.

(5 minute station)

Patient history	Biochemical abnormality	Diagnosis
1 A 64-year-old man with a known small-cell carcinoma and cerebral metastases	(A) Na$^+$ 121 K$^+$ 6.7 Glucose 21.3 CCa^{2+} 1.98 Ur 56.8 Cr 1098	(a) Hypomagnesaemia
2 A 32-year-old woman two days post-parathyroidectomy	(B) Na$^+$ 134 K$^+$ 3.7 Glucose 1.2 CCa^{2+} 2.43 Ur 2.3 Cr 67	(b) Decompensated hepatic failure
3 A 49-year-old man on high doses of frusemide	(C) Na$^+$ 123 Glucose 3.8 K$^+$ 3.4 Albumin 23 Ur 1.9 AST 435 Cr 49 Alk phos 598 Bili 43	(c) Hypoglycaemia
4 A 34-year-old man with end-stage renal failure secondary to diabetic nephropathy	(D) Na$^+$ 103 Glucose 6.4 K$^+$ 3.9 CCa^{2+} 2.56 Ur 8.9 Mg^{2+} 0.69 Cr 108	(d) Hypocalcaemia
5 A 41-year-old alcohol abuser who presents with confusion and melaena	(E) Na$^+$ 141 Glucose 5.7 K$^+$ 4.0 CCa^{2+} 1.38 Ur 5.9 Mg^{2+} 0.73 Cr 123	(e) SIADH
6 A 59-year-old individual with NIDDM controlled on gliclazide tablets	(F) Na$^+$ 136 Glucose 4.6 K$^+$ 4.9 CCa^{2+} 2.08 Ur 6.1 Mg^{2+} 0.42 Cr 76	(f) Uraemia

Answers

1 (   ) (   )   5 (   ) (   )

2 (   ) (   )   6 (   ) (   )

3 (   ) (   )

4 (   ) (   )

STATION 2.21

Investigation

Please answer the questions below about the three CSF samples A, B and C. The normal values are shown for comparison.

(5 minute station)

CSF	Normal values	Sample (A)	Sample (B)	Sample (C)
Appearance	Clear	Turbid	Clear	Turbid/purulent
Mononuclear (cells/mm^3)	<5	290	57	12
Polymorph (cells/mm^3)	Nil	180	Nil	2460
Protein (g/l)	0.2–0.4 >0.5	2.63 <0.33	0.67 >0.5	1.55 <0.33
Glucose	plasma glucose	plasma glucose	plasma glucose	plasma glucose

Please indicate the correct answers by ticking the appropriate boxes.
There may be more than one correct answer per question.

	A	B	C
1 Which of the patient(s) should have contact tracing?	☐	☐	☐
2 Which patient(s) must receive antibiotic therapy?	☐	☐	☐
3 Which patient(s) should be nursed in a dark, quiet room?	☐	☐	☐
4 Which patient is most likely to present in DIC?	☐	☐	☐
5 Which of the patient(s) is most likely to be from the Indian subcontinent?	☐	☐	☐
6 Which patient(s) may have significantly raised ASO titres?	☐	☐	☐
7 Which patient(s) may have significant changes on their CXR?	☐	☐	☐

	A	B	C
8 Which patients are most likely to suffer with hydrocephalus?	☐	☐	☐
9 Which patient(s) will have a clear Gram stain?	☐	☐	☐
10 Which patient(s) may have a positive Kernig's sign?	☐	☐	☐

STATION 2.22

Investigation

Please match the patient histories with the correct diagnosis and CSF findings.

(5 minute station)

Patient history	CSF	Diagnosis
1 23-year-old woman with painful blurring of vision and numbness in the hands	(A) Xanthochromia	(a) Meningococcal meningitis
2 A neonate with diarrhoea and vomiting, 'off feeds' and extreme irritability	(B) High red cell count in all three CSF bottles	(b) Tertiary syphilis
3 12-year-old schoolgirl with purpura, DIC and severe headache, photophobia and neck stiffness	(C) VDRL, TPHA, FTA positive	(c) Subarachnoid haemorrhage
4 78-year-old man with recurrent falls and confusion	(D) Raised protein Low glucose Gram-negative coccobacillus	(d) Multiple sclerosis
5 27-year-old woman with sudden onset of severe headache and coma	(E) Raised protein Low glucose Gram-negative diplococci	(e) Subdural haemorrhage
6 61-year-old woman with increasing confusion and a previous history of pelvic inflammatory disease	(F) Oligoclonal bands	(f) *Haemophilus influenzae* meningitis

Answers

1 (   ) (   )   4 (   ) (   )

2 (   ) (   )   5 (   ) (   )

3 (   ) (   )   6 (   ) (   )

STATION 2.23

Investigation

Please identify the labelled structures in these anteroposterior and lateral radiographs of a normal skull (figs 2.23a and 2.23b).

(5 minute station)

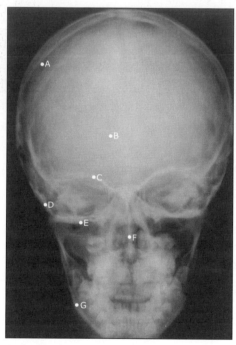

fig 2.23a

Answers

(A)   (E)

(B)   (F)

(C)   (G)

(D)

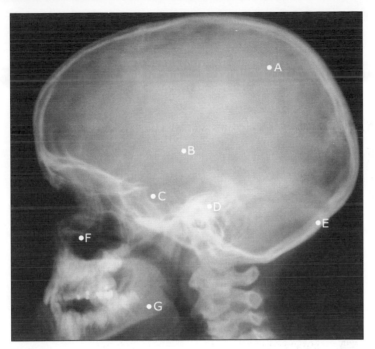

fig 2.23b

Answers

(A)

(B)

(C)

(D)

(E)

(F)

(G)

STATION 2.24

Investigation

Please indicate whether the statements regarding the three skull radiographs, figs 2.24a, 2.24b and 2.24c, shown below are **True** or **False**.

(5 minute station)

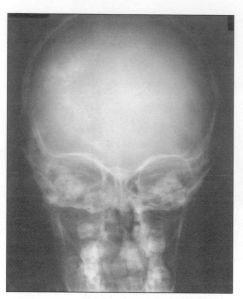 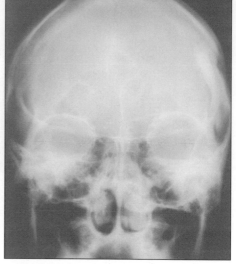

fig 2.24a   fig 2.24b

1 (fig 2.24a)	True	False
(a) This is an AP view of the skull	☐	☐
(b) The sinuses appear normal	☐	☐
(c) The cortex is normal	☐	☐
(d) There is evidence of intracerebral calcification	☐	☐
(e) The disorder shown is associated with seizures	☐	☐

2 (fig 2.24b)	True	False
(a) This is a lateral skull radiograph	☐	☐
(b) There is evidence of cortical thickening	☐	☐
(c) There is evidence of intracerebral calcification	☐	☐
(d) There is a depressed parietal fracture	☐	☐
(e) This patient requires surgical elevation of the fracture	☐	☐

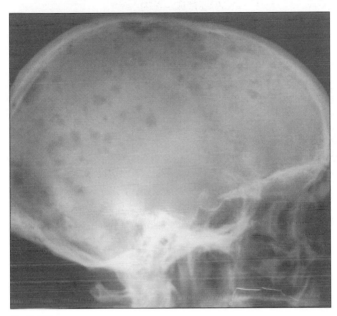

fig 2.24a

3 (fig 2.24c)	True	False
(a) This is a lateral skull radiograph	☐	☐
(b) The patient has multiple osteosclerotic lesions	☐	☐
(c) This patient will be expected to have hypocalcaemia	☐	☐
(d) The patient will have a paraproteinaemia	☐	☐
(e) This disorder is associated with amyloidosis	☐	☐

STATION 2.25

Investigation

Please identify the structures labelled below in the CT scans of the head shown in figs 2.25a and 2.25b.

(5 minute station)

(a) CT head scan – level of the orbits

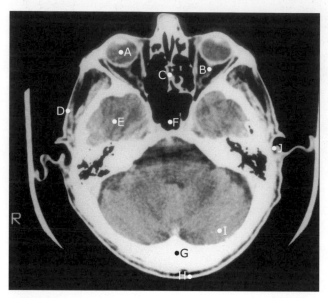

fig 2.25a

Answers

(A)

(B)

(C)

(D)

(E)

(F)

(G)

(H)

(I)

(J)

(b) CT head scan – level of the lateral ventricles

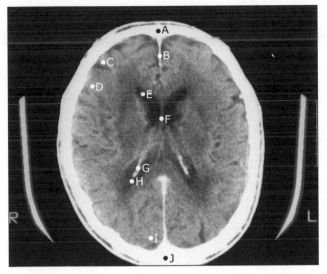

fig 2.25b

Answers

(A)

(B)

(C)

(D)

(E)

(F)

(G)

(H)

(I)

(J)

STATION 2.26

Investigation

Please indicate whether the statements regarding the three CT head scans shown in figs 2.26a, 2.26b and 2.26c are **True** or **False**.

(5 minute station)

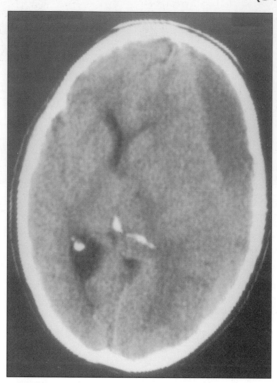

fig 2.26a

1 (*fig 2.26a*)	True	False
(a) The patient should be given warfarin	☐	☐
(b) The patient has hydrocephalus	☐	☐
(c) There is evidence of midline shift	☐	☐
(d) There is an extradural haemorrhage	☐	☐
(e) The patient requires neurosurgical intervention	☐	☐

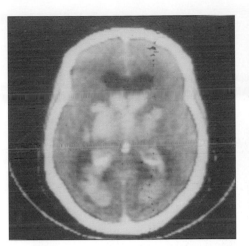

fig 2.26b

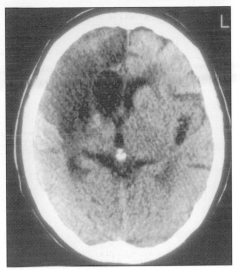

fig 2.26c

2 (fig 2.26b)	True	False
(a) The scan shows interventricular blood	☐	☐
(b) The headache associated with this disorder is classically insidious in onset	☐	☐
(c) Xanthochromia is a feature of delayed lumbar puncture in this disorder	☐	☐
(d) The patient should always have neurosurgical intervention	☐	☐
(e) The patient should receive nimodipine	☐	☐

3 (fig 2.26c)	True	False
(a) The patient will have a right-sided extensor plantar response	☐	☐
(b) The patient is likely to be hypertensive on admission	☐	☐
(c) There is evidence of a left occipital infarct	☐	☐
(d) There is evidence of midline shift	☐	☐
(e) The prognosis in this case will be improved by dipyridamole SR therapy	☐	☐

STATION 2.27

Investigation

Please indicate whether the statements below regarding the investigations (figs 2.27a, 2.27b, 2.27c and 2.27d) are **True** or **False**.

(5 minute station)

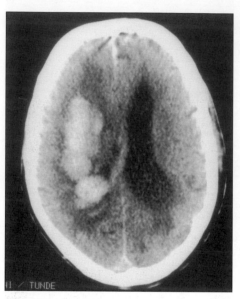

fig 2.27a

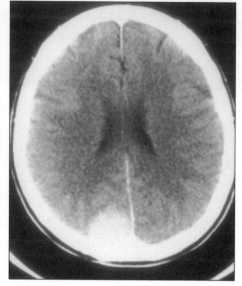

fig 2.27b

1 (fig 2.27a)	True	False
(a) This is a CT scan with contrast	☐	☐
(b) There is evidence of hydrocephalus	☐	☐
(c) There is evidence of midline shift	☐	☐
(d) This appearance is consistent with a primary malignant tumour	☐	☐
(e) This patient is a candidate for radiotherapy	☐	☐

2 (fig 2.27b)	True	False
(a) There is evidence of raised intracranial pressure	☐	☐
(b) The ventricles are normal	☐	☐
(c) This contrast-enhanced scan shows evidence of an intracranial haemorrhage	☐	☐
(d) This patient will be blind	☐	☐
(e) This patient is a candidate for neurosurgery	☐	☐

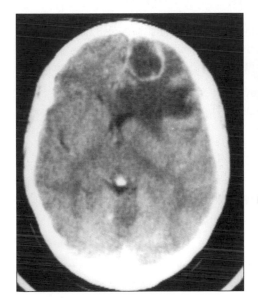

fig 2.27c

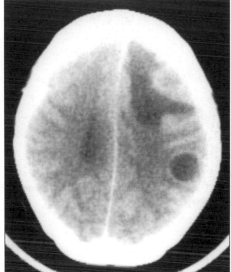

fig 2.27d

3 (fig 2.27c and fig 2.27d)	True	False
(a) There is evidence of cerebral oedema	☐	☐
(b) There is a frontal infarct	☐	☐
(c) There is a ring enhancing lesion	☐	☐
(d) There is evidence of midline shift	☐	☐
(e) This patient should receive nimodipine	☐	☐

STATION 2.28

Therapeutics: prepatory station

You have five minutes to read the information shown below before attempting the next station.

(5 minute station)

You are a house officer in the outpatient clinic of a specialist neurology firm. The next patient is a 23-year-old fashion model who was diagnosed as having epilepsy six months ago. Since then she has been having increasingly frequent fits, with six or seven in the last two weeks. She lives a very hectic life because of her work and she claims that she 'needs' to drive a car (which she is still doing). She is on no medications other than the oral contraceptive pill. She drinks 20 to 30 units of alcohol per week but occasionally drinks a lot more at parties. She also admits to occasionally using recreational drugs, including cannabis and cocaine. She is very keen to accept any help with stopping her fits but is reluctant to take medications.

Please discuss the possible changes she may need to make to her lifestyle, and the pros and cons of drug therapy for her epilepsy. After reading this information, please continue with the next station.

STATION 2.28a

Therapeutics

The patient in the outpatient clinic is the 23-year-old fashion model with poorly controlled epilepsy. Please discuss the lifestyle changes that she may need to make to help with her control, and the pros and cons of starting drug therapy.

(10 minute station)

STATION 2.29

Treatment

Please match the patient history with the correct diagnosis and therapy.

(5 minute station)

Patient history	Diagnosis	Therapy
1 A 24-year-old man with parasthesiae of his hands and feet and painful blurring of his vision	(A) Alzheimer's disease	(a) Selegiline and L-dopa
2 An 18-year-old woman with exertional weakness and a thymoma	(B) Normal pressure hydrocephalus	(b) Prednisolone
3 A 71-year-old man with a festenating gait and a resting tremor	(C) Multiple sclerosis	(c) Donepezil
4 A 63-year-old man with progressive confusion and disability	(D) Myasthenia gravis	(d) Ventriculo-peritoneal shunt
5 A 43-year-old woman with angina, jaw claudication and headaches	(E) Parkinson's disease	(e) Physostigmine
6 A 79-year-old man with increasing confusion, gait dyspraxia and urinary incontinence	(F) Giant cell arteritis	(f) Beta interferon

Answers

1 (   ) (   )
2 (   ) (   )
3 (   ) (   )
4 (   ) (   )
5 (   ) (   )
6 (   ) (   )

STATION 2.30

Procedure: consent for lumbar puncture

You are the medical house officer attached to a general medical firm. You have been asked by the registrar to gain consent for a lumbar puncture from a 23-year-old woman with a poorly resolving headache. A CT head scan was unremarkable and she has no papilloedema. Please obtain verbal consent for the procedure and answer any questions she may have.

(5 minute station)

STATION 2.31

History

You are a medical student attached to a psychiatry firm. The next patient in the outpatient clinic is a 43-year-old woman who has been referred by her GP with 'feeling very low'. Please take a history of the presenting complaint and any relevant history with a view to making a diagnosis.

(10 minute station)

STATION 2.32

History

You are a medical student attached to a psychiatry firm. You have been asked by the duty psychiatrist to clerk a patient in the Emergency Department. The patient is a 23-year-old man who has been brought in by his family after several episodes of 'very strange behaviour'. Please take a history of the presenting complaint and any further relevant history with a view to making a diagnosis.

(10 minute station)

STATION 2.33

History

You are a house officer attached to a general medical firm. You have been asked to see a patient in the Emergency Department who has been referred after trying to kill herself. Please assess this patient's suicidal intent with a view to admitting her to hospital.

(10 minute station)

STATION 2.34

History

You are a medical student attached to a GP practice. A patient has come to see the doctor about a 'private matter concerning her husband'. She has agreed to talk to you. Please take a history of the presenting complaint and any other relevant history with a view to making a diagnosis.

(10 minute station)

STATION 2.35

History

You are a house officer attached to an alcohol dependency unit as part of your psychiatry attachment. The next patient is a 43-year-old football manager who has been referred by his GP for alcohol detoxification. Please take a history of his alcohol abuse and any other relevant history with a view to admitting him onto the detoxification programme.

(5 minute station)

STATION 2.36

History

You are a medical student attached to a GP practice. The next patient is a 27-year-old woman who has come to see the doctor because she cannot stop washing her hands. Please take a history of the presenting complaint and any other relevant history, with a view to making a diagnosis.

(5 minute station)

STATION 2.37

History

You are the medical house officer on call. You have been called to see a 72-year-old woman, who is demanding to go home, despite the fact it is 3 o'clock in the morning. Please assess this patient's mental state and decide whether she can be allowed to go home. A routine set of observations has recently been performed by the nursing staff.

(5 minute station)

STATION 2.38

Investigation

The following patients have presented with acute confusion. Please match the histories with the most appropriate diagnosis and investigation results.

(5 minute station)

Patient history	Investigations		Diagnosis
1 A 39-year-old alcohol abuser with liver flap and jaundice	(A) Na$^+$ 122 K$^+$ 6.1 Ur 9.6 Cr 135	Albumin 36 CCa^{2+} 2.45 Glucose 3.2 Bili 14	(a) End-stage renal failure
2 A 56-year-old man with known metastatic carcinoma of the lung	(B) Na$^+$ 126 K$^+$ 6.9 Ur 67 Cr 1067	Albumin 13 Bili 12 CCa^{2+} 1.98 Glucose 4.8	(b) Diabetic ketoacidosis
3 A 24-year-old woman with polydypsia polyuria and a chest infection	(C) Na$^+$ 125 K$^+$ 3.4 Ur 1.9 Cr 67	Albumin 23 Bili 48 Glucose 3.8	(c) SIADH secondary to *Legionella pneumophila*
4 A 49-year-old woman on long-term steroids for polymyalgia rheumatica, presenting with three days of vomiting	(D) Na$^+$ 115 K$^+$ 4.3 Ur 5.6 Cr 67	Albumin 38 CCa^{2+} 2.38 PO^{4-} 0.36 Glucose 5.9	(d) Ectopic parathyroid-like hormone production
5 A 34-year-old woman with peripheral oedema, shortness of breath, a flap and 'frosted' skin	(E) Na$^+$ 139 K$^+$3.6 Ur 12 Cr 123	Albumin 31 CCa^{2+} 2.17 Glucose 45.7	(e) Addisonian crisis
6 A 27-year-old woman who has just returned from holiday in Spain, presenting with dry cough and diarrhoea	(F) Na$^+$ 124 K$^+$ 4.6 Ur 3.9 Cr 124	Albumin 29 CCa^{2+} 4.31 PO4- 0.58 Glucose 4.9	(f) Hepatic encephalopathy

Answers

1 (   ) (   )
2 (   ) (   )
3 (   ) (   )
4 (   ) (   )
5 (   ) (   )
6 (   ) (   )

STATION 2.39

Investigation

You are a medical student attached to a psychiatry firm. Over the weekend several of the inpatients have become acutely confused. Please match the patient histories with the most appropriate investigation and diagnosis.

(5 minute station)

Patient history	Investigation	Diagnosis
1 A 29-year-old schizophrenic recently started on new treatment. Now he is rigid and has a temperature of 41°C	(A) Na^+ 119 CCa^{2+} 4.02 K^+ 3.9 Ur 3.8 Cr 78	(a) Lithium toxicity
2 A 69-year-old being investigated for recent aggressive behaviour and change in personality	(B) Na^+ 112 CCa^{++} 2.64 K^+ 4.2 Ur 4.2 Cr 102	(b) Delirium tremens
3 A 31-year-old manic depressive with polyuria	(C) Na^+ 134 Hb 11.4 K^+ 5.0 MCV 108 Ur 1.6 WCC 4.3 Cr 78 Plats 64	(c) SSRI induced hyponatraemia
4 A 41-year-old alcohol abuser admitted for alcohol withdrawal	(D) Na^+ 153 K^+ 3.6 Ur 5.8 Cr 112	(d) Neuroleptic malignant syndrome
5 A 77-year-old demented woman with depression	(E) Na^+ 142 CK 2067 K^+ 4.7 Ur 12.2 Cr 135	(e) SIADH secondary to metastatic carcinoma of the lung

Answers

1 ( ) ( )
2 ( ) ( )
3 ( ) ( )
4 ( ) ( )
5 ( ) ( )
6 ( ) ( )

STATION 2.40

Investigation

You are the medical student attached to a psychogeriatric firm. The patients below have been labelled as having dementia. Please match the patient histories with the most appropriate investigation and diagnosis.

(5 minute station)

Patient history	Investigation	Diagnosis
1 A 69-year-old man with hypertension and several strokes and MIs in the past	(A) TSH 22.5 fT4 3.5	(a) Creutzfeldt-Jakob disease
2 A 79-year-old man with ataxia, confusion and urinary incontinence	(B) CCa^{2+} 1.57	(b) Neurosyphilis (GPI)
3 An 83-year-old woman with slow relaxing reflexes and a husky voice	(C) CT head – multiple small infarcts	(c) Subacute combined degeneration of the cord
4 A 77-year-old man with weakness in the lower limbs, hyporeflexia and a previous history of treponemal disease	(D) CSF – prion protein identified by PCR	(d) Hypo-parathyroidism
5 A 70-year-old woman with anaemia, peripheral neuropathy and leg weakness	(E) CT head scan – grossly dilated ventricles; CSF opening pressure =10 cm	(e) Multi-infarct dementia
6 A 78-year-old man with ataxia, seizures and rapidly progressive confusion	(F) B_{12} 2.7 Folate:15	(f) Hypothyroidism

7 A 69-year-old woman with insidious worsening confusion and tetany

(G) CSF – FTA/TPHA positive

(g) Normal pressure hydrocephalus

Answers

1 (   ) (   )
2 (   ) (   )
3 (   ) (   )
4 (   ) (   )
5 (   ) (   )
6 (   ) (   )
7 (   ) (   )

STATION 2.41

Therapeutics

Please read the following information before attempting the next station.

(5 minute station)

You are the medical student attached to a psychiatry firm. The registrar has asked you to explain to a relatively well controlled schizophrenic about depot injections for the administration of his antipsychotic medication. He has left you the following information to relay to the patient.

Reasons to change from tablets: after initial adjustments it will mean only one injection every 2–4 weeks instead of daily tablets. Depot injections often increase compliance, which in turn improves control.

What it involves: initially a small test dose is given to ensure no adverse effects.

- If this is successful then injections are given with a slow reduction in tablets
- Regular deep intramuscular injections are given every 2–4 weeks
- Injections are 2–3 ml of oily solution
- Injection sites are rotated to reduce local side-effects

Side-effects

- Local: pain, bruising, swelling, erythema, nodules
- Systemic: increase Parkinsonian and extrapyramidal symptoms

Caution: response to treatment is variable and may require several months of adjustment of the dose before a suitable regime is found.

STATION 2.41a

Therapeutics

The patient in the outpatient clinic is the relatively well-controlled schizophrenic who would like to go on depot injections for his antipsychotic medication. Please explain the treatment to him.

(5 minute station)

STATION 2.42

Therapeutics

Please match the medications with the most appropriate investigation and side-effect

(5 minute station)

Medication	Investigation	Side-effect
1 Lithium	(A) WCC 2.1	(a) Galactorrhoea
2 Fluoxetine	(B) CK 3078	(b) Cholestatic jaundice
3 Amitriptyline	(C) Pyridoxine levels grossly reduced	(c) SIADH
4 Haloperidol	(D) Prolactin 934	(d) Agranulocytosis
5 Chlorpromazine	(E) TSH 25.6 fT4 2.4	(e) Peripheral neuropathy
6 Phenelzine	(F) Na^+ 112	(f) Neuroleptic malignant syndrome
7 Flupenthixol	(G)AST 434 Alk phos 621 Bili 43	(g) Hypothyroidism

Answers

1 (   ) (   )
2 (   ) (   )
3 (   ) (   )
4 (   ) (   )
5 (   ) (   )
6 (   ) (   )
7 (   ) (   )

Chapter 3:
Ophthalmology and
Otolaryngology

Contents

Chapter 3

Ophthalmology and Otolaryngology

Ophthalmology History

The eye is affected in many local and systemic diseases and is a sensitive monitor of their progress, since relatively mild disease can produce severe loss of function. The healing process itself can interfere with vision, as revascularisation and scarring can opacify vital optically clear tissues. The retina and optic nerve are derivatives of the central nervous system and do not regenerate.

Disease may affect all or part of the ocular apparatus; examples of the former are trauma and infection. Trauma includes physical and chemical agents, and systemic toxins; the latter includes lead, arsenic, insecticides, and some antibiotics and antimalarial agents. Infection may be limited to the conjunctiva but extension into the globe can cause perforation, and the aqueous and vitreous humours are good culture media. Systemic diseases affecting the eye include thyrotoxicosis, diabetic retinopathy and a number of autoimmune conditions, producing scleritis and iridocyclitis. These include rheumatoid arthritis, inflammatory bowel disease, sarcoid, Reiter's syndrome and ankylosing spondylitis. The lens may opacify with age, dislocation occurring in Marfan's disease. Tumours may involve the globe or the retro-orbital tissues.

Eye symptoms include abnormalities of vision, abnormal appearance and pain. The problem may be uni- or bilateral, and focal or general.

Abnormalities of vision

Congenital abnormalities
Congenital abnormalities include myopic, hypermetropic and defective colour vision, changing acuity with age. Blurring of vision may be due to infection and inflammation of any part of the globe.

Retinal abnormalities
Examples of retinal abnormalities are diabetic retinopathy, hypertension, papilloedema and increased ocular pressure as in glaucoma. Glaucoma may produce a halo around objects, as well as blurring of the vision.

Loss of vision
This occurs in neurological abnormalities of the optic nerve and tract: pituitary tumours produce bitemporal hemianopia; lesions of the tract and cortex produce a homonomous hemianopia. Optic nerve damage may be due to trauma and optic neuritis, as in multiple sclerosis.

Vascular abnormalities
These can give rise to ischaemia of the retina or the optic nerve, as in central artery or central venous thrombosis. Emboli from sites such as the carotid bifurcation produce amaurosis fugax, and untreated giant cell arteritis can produce blindness.

Abnormal appearances

The eyelid becomes **oedematous**, due to infection of the conjunctiva and orbital cellulitis. Local blockage of glands or follicles may produce infection or cysts, such as a stye or chalazion. Protrusion of the eyeball (**exophthalmos**) is found in thyroid eye disease, ocular and orbital tumours, caroticocavernous fistulae and carotid sinus thrombosis. Thyroid eye disease also produces upper and lower lid retraction, lid lag, nystagmus and, in severe cases, conjunctivitis and exophthalmic ophthalmoplegia, often accompanied by diplopia. Horner's syndrome produces **enophthalmos**, **myosis** and **loss of sweating** on the ipsilateral face.

Entropion and **ectropion** produce discomfort and associated conjunctival infection. Blockage of lachrymal drainage can produce discomfort, discharge and local swelling, sometimes with an associated mucocoele. A **squint** may be congenital or secondary to ocular or cerebral damage and accompanied by diplopia. A defective iris may be congenital (coloboma) or acquired in the treatment of glaucoma. Wide **dilatation** of the pupil can be due to damage of the optic nerve and ocular pathways, and the pupil may be non-responsive. It may also be due to atropine-like drugs. Small pupils can be linked with opiates and may be irregular in tabes dorsalis. An intra-ocular tumour can alter the normal red eye reflex, a typical white or yellow **cat's eye** reflex being observed in children with retinoblastoma.

The conjunctiva may be stained **yellow** in jaundice: **red eye** is most commonly due to conjunctivitis but is also associated with trauma, infection and inflammation within the eye, raised intra-ocular pressure and retro-orbital disease. Conjunctivitis is produced by a wide variety of organisms, as well as allergy, trauma, chemicals and ultraviolet light. Infection is associated with oedematous **swelling** and **discharge**. This may be inflammatory with lacrimation, the patient complaining of a gritty feeling within the eye, and sticky eyelids.

Itchiness

Itchiness is associated with conjunctival infection and is present in allergic and bacterial conjunctivitis.

Pain

Pain in the eye accompanies infection and trauma but is also a warning sign in glaucoma, uveitis and keratitis. Pain is often accompanied by **photophobia**.

Ophthalmology Examination

Examination of the eye and orbit

Compare the appearances of the two sides. Assess visual acuity, eg counting fingers at three feet, or Snellen and colour vision charts.

- **Eyelids:** injury/oedema, discharge, deformity, ptosis, lid lag or retraction
- **Orbital rim:** palpate for the presence of a fracture
- **Globe:** examine for any displacement (exophthalmos, enophthalmos) and abnormal ocular movement
- **Pupil:** assess shape and pupillary reflex
- **Cornea:** use fluorescein and an ultraviolet light to examine for foreign bodies or abrasions
- **Conjunctiva:** examine for haemorrhage, chemosis and subconjunctival emphysema (indicating fracture of the orbit into an adjacent sinus), jaundice, anaemia
- **Anterior chamber:** examine for depth and for presence of hyphaema or foreign bodies
- **Iris:** examine for pupil shape, deformity or defect
- **Lens:** assess transparency and displacement or dislocation
- **Vitreous:** vitreous haemorrhage obscures normal transparency on fundoscopy, look for opacities and foreign bodies
- **Retina:** examine with an ophthalmoscope for haemorrhage, discoloration, tears or detachment, papilloedema and vessel pattern, size, nipping, aneurysms and tumours

OSCE Stations

Otolaryngology History

Ears

As with all causes of pain, the character including site, radiation, onset, duration, severity, and exacerbating and relieving factors needs to be defined.

Causes of pain

- **External ear**
  Injury, haematoma of the pinna
  Otitis externa, bacterial or fungal
  Perichondritis – rare
- **Middle ear**
  Acute suppurative otitis media, principally *Streptococcus* and *Haemophilus* infections
  Chronic secretory otitis media – 'glue ear'
  Acute mastoiditis
- **Referred pain**
  Derived from structures sharing a common innervation with the ear. These include oro and laryngopharynx – tonsillitis, carcinoma
  Teeth – upper molars, impacted wisdom teeth, poor-fitting dentures
  Temporomandibular joint
  Parotid swelling
  Cervical spondylosis (C2,3)

Associated symptoms

- Fever
- Upper respiratory tract symptoms
- Cervical lymphadenopathy

Discharge from the ear – otorrhoea

- Purulent or mucopurulent – often indicates acute otitis media
- Serous fluid – otitis externa
- Clear or blood-stained fluid after a head injury should be treated as a CSF leak until proven otherwise
- Smelly/offensive – cholesteatoma, associated deafness and vertigo

Hearing impairment/deafness

This severe disability leads to problems with communication and language. It is defined by rate of onset, age of onset, degree of impairment, uni- or bilateral ear involvement. Causes are divided into conductive and sensorineural.

OSCE Stations

- **Tinnitus:** the perception of hearing noises
  It is defined by – onset, duration, severity and character of the noise. It is often associated with hearing impairment
- **Vertigo**: the perception of movement either of the patient with respect to their surroundings, or vice versa. Patients often describe the feeling as 'being drunk'
  Defined by onset – acute, eg vestibular neuritis, trauma, vertebrobasilar ischaemia
  Postural change – benign postural vertigo
  Chronic – Ménière's disease, cholesteatoma

Associated symptoms
- Nausea and vomiting
- Auditory symptoms – tinnitus, deafness
- Central nervous causes have associated neurological symptoms (eg ataxia, dysarthria, diplopia)

Nose

Loss of smell – hypo/anosmia

Causes
- Smoking
- Coryza
- Cribriform plate fracture
- Frontal meningioma

Pain

By defining the character of the pain, the cause is usually obvious.

- **Acute/severe**
  Infection
  Trauma
- **Chronic/dull**
  Sinusitis (may become severe)
  Tumours of the nasal passage/sinuses

Discharge

- **Defined by – character**
  Bloody
  Mucopurulent
  Serous
  Clear – after trauma one should suspect CSF leak
- **Unilateral**
  Foreign body
  Tumour – carcinoma
  Polyps
  Post-nasal drip – discharge from the back of the nose into the oropharynx; can lead to an odd taste in the mouth and halitosis

Causes

- Infection
- Foreign body

Obstruction

Defined by uni- or bilateral involvement, permanent or intermittent.

Causes

- Allergic rhinitis
- Coryza
- Polyps
- Trauma
- Foreign body
- Tumour

Bleeding – epistaxis

Causes

- **Trauma**
  Iatrogenic, accidental
  Spontaneous/idiopathic <30 years old – common: anterior septum (Little's area). >30 years old – less common: posterior septum
- **Tumours**
  Benign – polyps, angiofibroma
  Malignant: carcinoma – nasal sinuses
  Lymphoma
  Miscellaneous
  Wegener's granulomatosis
- **Hereditary haemorrhagic telangiectasia**
  (Osler–Weber–Rendu syndrome)
- **Hypertension**
- **Coagulopathy**
- **Iatrogenic**
  Warfarin
  Heparin

Throat

Hoarseness

Partial loss of the voice may lead to complete voice loss; prolonged hoarseness should always be investigated.

Causes

- Acute/chronic laryngitis
- Recurrent laryngeal nerve-palsy
- Vocal cord (glottic); supra- and subglottic carcinoma

Stridor

Obstruction of the upper respiratory tract leads to difficulty in breathing and 'whistling/wheezing' breath sounds.

Causes

- Acute epiglottitis
- Trauma
- Large goitre
- Upper respiratory tract tumours

Dysphagia

- The feeling of food or liquid sticking within the oropharynx or oesophagus
- Defined by – level: oropharynx, upper, mid, lower oesophagus

Associated symptoms

- Aspiration
- Regurgitation
- Dysarthria

Causes

- Neuromuscular disorders
- Motor neurone disease
- Poliomyelitis
- Syringobulbia
- Brainstem CVA
- Multiple sclerosis
- Pharyngeal pouch
- Large goitre
- Benign/malignant strictures of the oesophagus.
- Achalasia of the cardia

Otolarygology Examination

The external ear

This consists of examination of the external ear, the auditory meatus and the eardrum. The external meatus is swabbed clear of wax, discharge or blood before auroscopic inspection of the meatal walls and the drum. Foreign bodies in the meatus may be identified and removed. The characteristics of the drum (ie tears, tension, discoloration, may indicate middle ear disease).

The nose and nasopharynx

Anterior rhinoscopy: the tip of the nose is turned upwards and backwards by the examiner's thumb and a nasal speculum is introduced in adults. Structures visualised are: floor of nose, inferior and middle turbinates (and meati) and septum (superior turbinates are not visible).

Posterior rhinoscopy: performed with a postnasal mirror or by fibrescope. Structures visualised are: posterior aspects of middle and inferior turbinates, posterior edge of nasal septum and orifices of eustachian tubes.

The oropharynx

With a tongue depressor the following are visualised:

- Anterior faucial pillars (colour changes, ulceration or scarring)
- Tonsils (size, mobility, prescence of pus, debris and concretions)
- Tonsilolingual sulcus (important site for tumour growths) lies between tonsil and base of tongue
- Lateral laryngeal bands (for enlargement)
- Posterior pharyngeal wall (for swelling or ulceration)
- Movemenrs of the palate (on phonation and retching)

The laryngopharynx

By indirect laryngoscopy or fibrescopy the following are visualised:

- Base of tongue (lingual thyroid) and posterior and lateral walls of laryngopharynx
- Valleculae and laryngeal inlet (aryepiglottic folds and arytenoids, false and true cords – look for asymmetry, irregularity of edges, nodule formation, ulceration)
- Pyriform fossa and postcricord region (swelling, ulceration)

OSCE Stations

The cervical lymph nodes

In all age groups lymph node enlargement is the commonest lump in the neck, usually being of inflammatory origin particularly in the young. An important differential diagnosis is congenital anomalies, eg cystic hygroma, brachial cysts and carotid body tumours; if the latter is not considered, and biopsied, it can produce severe haemorrhage and inadvertent ligation of the internal carotid artery which may end with severe stroke or death.

In the elderly, progressive firm enlargement of a node is likely to be secondary neoplasia, examples being supraclavicular nodes from abdominal, bronchial and breast primaries, and a node around the base of the skull from the ear, nose or throat. Goitres are considered elsewhere but may also present or be accompanied by secondary lymph node enlargement. Diagnosis can usually be made on a fine needle aspirate of the node using ultrasound guidance.

Lymph nodes are sited as a ring around the base of the skull of named submental, submandibular, parotid, postauricular and occipital groups, and superficial (along the course of the external and anterior) or deep (internal jugular veins). The deep nodes may be sited in the retropharyngeal plane or around the digastric and omohyoid muscles, or be placed more laterally behind the sternomastoid and in the supraclavicular region.

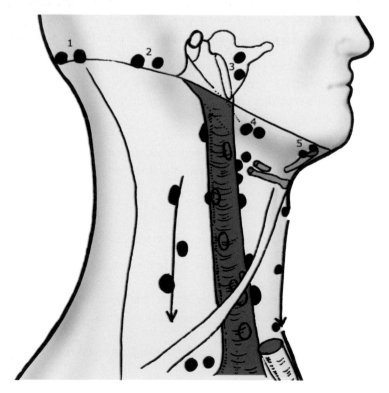

fig 3a

Anterior nodes are more easily palpable by examining the patient from behind and lateral nodes can be made more prominent by gently pressing the larynx towards the palpated side. Turning the chin against resistance tenses the sternomastoid on the examined side, helping to differentiate whether a lymph node is superficial, deep or tethered to the muscle.

Before starting to examine any neck lump, the patient should be asked how long they have had it, whether the lump is changing in size and, particularly, whether it is tender. If it is not obvious, also ask the patient to point out its situation.

As with all lumps, the examinee should have a list of features (that are consciously used during the examination rather than just recited). These include:

- Site, size, shape, surface, colour, temperature, tenderness, mobility
- Interior: consistency, compressibility, reducibility, cough impulse, fluid, thrill, indentation, fluctuation, discharge, pulsation, expansion, transillumination, bruit
- The surroundings: induration, tethering, invasion of the nerves, vessels, other tissues, nodes and related diseases

The examiner will usually request you to 'examine the lump in this patient's neck'. With generalised lymphatic disease, eg leukaemia and lymphoma, clinical examination is extended into the upper limb along the infraclavicular, axillary and epitrochlear nodes, and into the horizontal and vertical inguinal lymph nodes. There may be hepatosplenomegally and large para-aortic nodes may be palpable, but thoracic and abdominal lesions are best identified by imaging techniques.

OSCE Stations

STATION 3.1 *(Answers – page 303)*

History

A 13-year-old boy presents to you, a GP trainee, with inflamed, red and watering eyes. Please take a history and suggest the most likely diagnosis.

(5 minute station)

STATION 3.2

Examination

Please match the causes of a red eye with the most appropriate symptoms, disorder and disease marker.

(5 minute station)

Eye disorder	Symptoms	Systemic disorder	Systemic disease marker
1 Keratoconjunct-ivitis sicca	(A) Sticky discharge in itchy red eye, redness of both the eye and inside lids	(a) Rheumatoid arthritis	(F) Icosahedral DNA virus
2 Anterior uveitis/ iritis	(B) Severe pain with intense redness, occasionally bluish eye	(b) *Herpes simplex* virus	(G) Shigella infection
3 Bacterial conjunctivitis	(C) Pain, photophobia, watering, sectorial redness	(c) Reiter's syndrome	(H) aRo and aLa
4 Scleritis	(D) Dry, discomfort	(d) Ankylosing spondylitis	(I) IgM against IgG
5 Keratitis	(E) Pericorneal pain and photophobia, visible corneal precipitates	(e) Sjögren's syndrome	(J) HLA B27

Answers

1 (   ) (   )   4 (   ) (   )
2 (   ) (   )   5 (   ) (   )
3 (   ) (   )

STATION 3.3

History

A 42-year-old man presents to the Emergency Department complaining of pain in his left eye. Please take a history from this patient with a view to making a diagnosis.

(5 minute station)

STATION 3.4

Examination

The four figures (Figs 3.4a–3.4d) show eye conditions following blunt trauma.

(5 minute station)

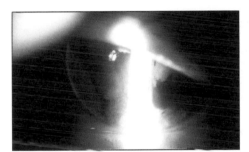

fig 3.4a

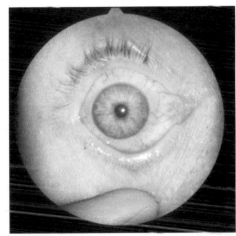

fig 3.4b

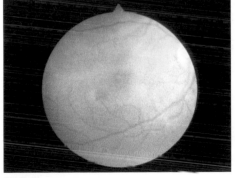

fig 3.4c

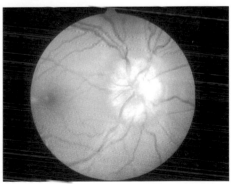

fig 3.4d

1 Please name the injury-induced pathology in each of the illustrations.

2 Please list eight other ocular injuries caused by blunt trauma.

3 Please tick the correct response to the following.

You would identify an intra-ocular foreign body by:

	True	False
(a) Ophthalmological examination.	☐	☐
(b) Fluorescein staining of the conjunctiva.	☐	☐
(c) Radiograph of the orbit.	☐	☐
(d) Ultrasonography of the orbit.	☐	☐
(e) Presence of intraocular haematoma.	☐	☐

STATION 3.5

Examination

Refer to the figs 3.5a–3.5d which relate to the following questions.

(5 minute station)

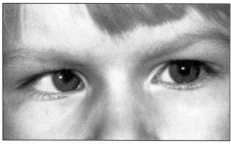

fig 3.5a. What is the diagnosis in this nine-year-old boy? How would you initially correct this condition?

fig 3.5a

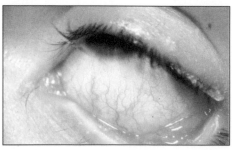

fig 3.5b. What is the diagnosis in this 30-year-old man, who was exposed to chemical fumes in an industrial accident? How would you initially treat this condition?

fig 3.5b

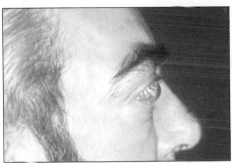

fig 3.5c

fig 3.5c. What is the diagnosis in this 58-year-old man? State two complications to the eye from this condition.

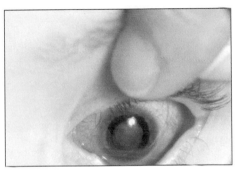

fig 3.5d

fig 3.5d. This is the eye of a seven-year-old boy. What is the probable diagnosis and a diagnostic feature that is demonstrated?

OSCE Stations

STATION 3.6

Examination

fig 3.6 shows a woman who complains of progressive visual symptoms.

(5 minute station)

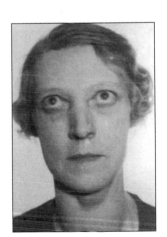

fig 3.6

1 What disease is affecting the eyes of this patient?

2 What is the associated eye condition called?

3 List three eye complications that may result.

4 How would you treat the eye lesion if it threatens vision?

STATION 3.7

Examination

fig 3.7a shows a painful swelling in the upper eyelid of a 21 year-old woman.
fig 3.7b shows a surgical instrument tray prepared to treat this lesion.

(5 minute station)

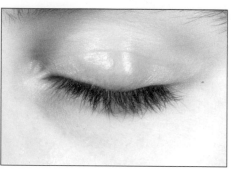

fig 3.7a

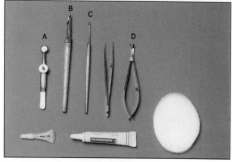

fig 3.7b

1 What is the diagnosis?

2 Name the items labelled in fig 3.7b to treat this condition.

(A)

(B)

(C)

(D)

3 How would you use these items in treating this lesion?

STATION 3.8

Examination

fig 3.8 shows the left eye of a 69-year-old man, who complained of failing vision on that side.

(5 minute station)

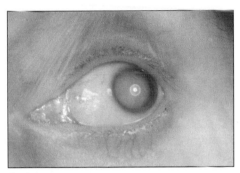

fig 3.8

1 What is the cause of his visual impairment?

2 List four predisposing causes of this condition.

3 State one absolute indication for treating this condition.

4 How would you treat this condition?

STATION 3.9

Examination

Please examine visual acuity and peripheral vision in this 25-year-old man (simulated patient). A Snellen chart (fig 3.9) is provided, please report your findings

(5 minute station)

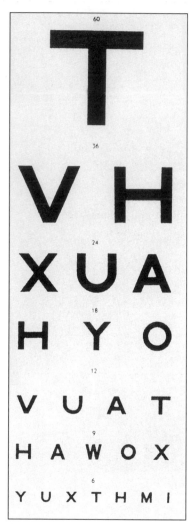

fig 3.9

STATION 3.10

Examination

Please match the eye signs with their associated inherited disorder and disease markers.

(5 minute station)

Eye disorder	Inherited disorder	Disease marker
1 Kayser–Fleischer rings	(A) Marfan's syndrome	(a) Glucocerebrocidase deficiency
2 Brushfield spots	(B) Tuberous sclerosis	(b) Yellowish reticulate plaques around the flexures
3 Superior dislocation of the lens	(C) Pseudoxanthoma elasticum	(c) Abnormal collagen gene
4 Pingueculae	(D) Wilson's disease	(d) TSC gene
5 Retinal phacoma	(E) Osteogenesis imperfecta	(e) Trisomy 21
6 Angioid streaks	(F) Tay–Sachs disease	(f) Abnormal fibrillin gene – chromosome 15
7 Macular cherry red spot	(G) Gaucher's disease	(g) Serum copper/ caeruloplasmin
8 Blue sclera	(H) Down's syndrome	(h) Hexosaminidase deficiency

Answers

1 (   ) (   )
2 (   ) (   )
3 (   ) (   )
4 (   ) (   )
5 (   ) (   )
6 (   ) (   )
7 (   ) (   )
8 (   ) (   )

OSCE Stations

STATION 3.11

History

You are a medical student attached to an ENT outpatient clinic. You have been asked to obtain a history from a 65-year-old man with a history of dizziness. Please take a history of the presenting complaint and any other relevant history with a view to making a diagnosis.

(5 minute station)

STATION 3.12

History

A 40-year-old woman is seen in the Emergency Department with a severe nose bleed. Please take a history with a view to making a diagnosis.

(5 minute station)

STATION 3.13

History

A woman holidaying with her family in a coastal resort brings her five-year-old daughter to the Emergency Department complaining that the child is ill with pain in her throat. Please take a history with a view to making a diagnosis.

(5 minute station)

STATION 3.14

Examination

(A) The patient in fig 3.14 has a facial abnormality.

(5 minute station)

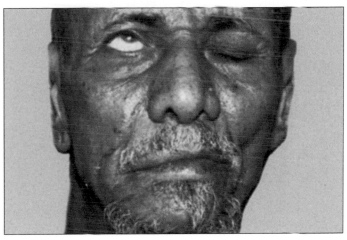

fig 3.14

1 What is the diagnosis?

2 How would you test for facial muscle weakness?

(B) Tick the appropriate column. Causes of facial palsy are:

	True	False
(a) Stroke	☐	☐
(b) Acoustic neuroma	☐	☐
(c) Polyneuritis	☐	☐
(d) Middle ear infection	☐	☐
(e) Parotid tumours	☐	☐
(f) Sarcoidosis	☐	☐
(g) Ear pain (may precede facial weakness in Bell's palsy)	☐	☐

(5 minute station)

STATION 3.15

Examination

The swelling on this patient's face (fig 3.15) is asymptomatic and has been present for five years.

(5 minute station)

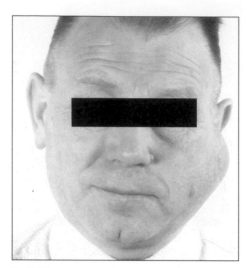

fig 3.15

1 What is the probable diagnosis and the pathological features of the swelling?

2 How would you treat this condition?

3 Please name a significant complication of treatment, and state how you would avoid this.

4 What would be the likely diagnosis if facial pain or facial palsy were a recent feature of the swelling?

STATION 3.16

History

A three-year-old boy with fever and pain in his ear is brought by his foster-mother to the GP surgery to see you, a GP trainee. Please take a history with a view to making a diagnosis.

(5 minute station)

STATION 3.17

Examination

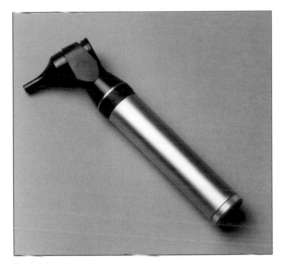

fig 3.17

You are a medical student attached to the ENT clinic. The next patient is a 25-year-old man with recent onset of hearing difficulties of the right side. Please examine his right ear with the instrument provided.

(5 minute station)

STATION 3.18

Examination

You are a medical student attached to a surgical firm. The next patient has been referred by his GP with 'a lump in the neck'. Please assess the lump with a view to making a diagnosis.

(5 minute station)

Chapter 4:
Urology and
Renal Medicine

Contents

Urogenital History

Assessment of the Renal Patient

Chapter 4

Urology and Renal Medicine

Urogenital History

- **Dysuria:** pain on passing urine – often described as a burning or stinging sensation
- **Strangury**: sudden painful cessation of micturition usually caused by vesical or urethral calculi
- **Frequency**: the number of times the bladder is emptied during the day and night (D/N)
- **Nocturia** the passing of urine at night
- **Haematuria:** may be blood mixed with the urine or frank blood. It is also important to define whether it is painful or painless. Painless haematuria should always be regarded as 'sinister' till proven otherwise
- **Incontinence:** may be stress or urge; may be a feature of infection if acute in onset
- **Prostatism:** symptoms of prostatic enlargement include hesitancy, frequency, poor urinary stream, terminal dribbling, incomplete evacuation and double micturition
- **Abdominal pain:** suprapubic – implies cystitis: loin pain ± radiation to groin – sharp, severe or spasmodic implies renal colic: dull, non-specific loin pain may occur due to renal cyst or tumour enlargement
- **Polyuria:** passing large volumes of urine; may be associated with polydypsia (increased thirst and fluid intake). It is a sign of diabetes mellitus or diabetes insipidus
- **Cloudy/offensive urine:** this is a sign of stagnation of the urine within the renal tract and often indicates infection. Patients on CAPD commonly present with 'cloudy' dialysate bags and abdominal pain when they are suffering with peritonitis secondary to their dialysis

Associated features

- Vaginal and penile discharge – other features of sexually transmitted diseases should be sought, with a full sexual history taken, including recent sexual contacts
- Fever/rigors – pyelonephritis is a common cause of rigors, shaking episodes secondary to fever. Renal cell carcinoma may present as a low grade fever and is a differential of a PUO
- Uraemia – confusion leading to coma, nausea and vomiting, pruritis, hiccoughs and pericarditis
- Peripheral oedema – is a sign of fluid overload and may be associated with ascites and symptoms of cardiac failure
- Systemic features of malignancy – weight loss, anorexia, malaise and fever
- Systemic features of hypertension – headaches and visual disturbance

Assessment of the Renal Patient

In OSCEs and more traditional clinical examinations the candidate is often simply invited to examine the patient's abdomen. You should always check for the signs listed below when instructions are quite simple and broad. Many candidates are caught out by always assuming the abdominal examination equates to examine for hepatosplenomegaly (never forget bimanual loin examination for the kidneys and the central abdomen for an abdominal aortic aneurysm).

When assessing the 'renal case' one must include/exclude:

1 Signs of dialysis

- Arterio-venous fistula (or PTFE graft)at the wrist or brachial
- Tenkoff catheter – in the anterior abdominal wall (CAPD catheter)
- Semi-permanent venous (tunnelled) catheter at neck, subclavian region or groin
- Scars from previous dialysis access in any of above regions

2 Signs of uraemia

- Metabolic flap/asterixis (whole body tremor)
- Uraemia pigmentation – in severe cases 'uraemic frost'
- Pruritis marks
- Confusion – associated with decreasing level of consciousness
- Hiccups

3 Signs of common underlying causes

- Diabetes – insulin pens; BM stix; BM chart; other complications (macro and microvascular; neurological)
- Polycystic kidney disease – enlarged kidneys
- Hypertension
- Generalised arteriopathy – signs of IHD, PVD and stroke
- Genetic syndromes – bilateral hearing aids, think patient with Alport's syndrome.

4 Signs of complications – acute and chronic renal failure

- Fluid overload – raised JVP; oedema; ascites; pleural effusions
- Nephrotic/nephritic – peripheral oedema; hypertension, facial oedema, ascites, pleural effusions
- Urinalysis
    - nephrotic – proteinuria^{+++}
    - nephritic – haematuria +/- proteinuria
    - diabetes mellitus - glycosuria +/- proteinuria
    - urinary tract infection – haematuria, proteinuria and nitrites

- Anaemia
- Indwelling urinary catheter, suprapubic catheter, nephrostomy tube

5   **Renal masses and scars**
- Unilateral/bilaterally enlarged kidneys
- Pelvic (transplanted) kidney
- Scars from previous transplants or native nephrectomies

In general – when considering the patient in renal failure

One: There is one cause of acute facial swelling – allergic reaction including anaphylaxis and angioneurotic oedema

Two: There are two, non-acute causes of facial and upper limb swelling. They are:
- Nephrotic syndrome
- Superior vena caval obstruction

Three: There are three causes of an enlarged kidney – they are:
- Hydronephrosis
- Benign tumours – eg cysts or abscesses
- Malignant tumours

Four: There are four life-threatening indications for emergency dialysis in a known dialysis patient; they are:
- Serum potassium >6.5 mmol/l
- Signs of fluid overload
- Worsening acidosis
- Pericardial rub and other signs of severe uraemia

STATION 4.1 *(Answers – page 327)*

History

You are a GP. The next patient is an 18-year old woman who is presenting with her fifth UTI in the past year. Please take a history of her urinary problems with a view to referring her to renal outpatients.

(5 minute station)

STATION 4.2

History

You are a medical student attached to a surgical firm. Please take a history from this 24-year-old patient with a view to making a diagnosis. You should be prepared to discuss the patient's management.

(5 minute station)

STATION 4.3

History

You are a medical house officer. You have been asked by your registrar to obtain a history from the wife of a confused patient who she is examining. Please take a history of the presenting complaint. You should be prepared to discuss the management options.

(5 minute station)

STATION 4.4

History

A 53-year-old man presents to urology outpatients with haematuria. You are the medical student attached to the firm. Please take a history of the presenting complaint with a view to making a diagnosis. You should be prepared to discuss the management of the patient.

(10 minute station)

OSCE Stations

STATION 4.5

History

You are the medical student attached to a general medical firm. Please take a history of the presenting complaint from the next patient who is a 37-year-old woman with systemic lupus erythematosus.

(5 minute station)

STATION 4.6

History

A 59-year-old woman sees you, her GP, with a complaint of urinary incontinence. Please take a history of the present complaint, and any other relevant factors, with a view to making a diagnosis.

(5 minute station)

STATION 4.7

Examination

Figs 4.7a–e depict five scrotal conditions listed in Table 4.7. The typical history, symptoms, signs and the treatment of each condition are arranged in a haphazard manner.

(5 minute station)

Condition	History	Symptoms	Signs	Treatment
1 Tesicular torsion	1a History of trauma	1b Painless scrotal swelling	1c swollen, red and tender scrotum with high transverse lie of testis	1d Repair of testicular injury
2 Varicoele	2a Enlarged testis	2b Painless testicular swelling	Swollen, red and tender with ecchymotic scrotum	2d Orchidectomy
3 Haematocele	3a Intermittant scrotal pain	3b Sharp onset of scrotal pain followed by swelling and redness	3c Cystic, non-tender scrotal swelling that trans-illuminates	3d Ligation of spermatic vein
4 Testicular tumour	4a Sub-fertility	4b Scrotal pain and swelling	4c Visible, palpable dilated veins above testis	4d excision or inversion of sac
5 Vaglnal hydrocele	5a Slow enlargement	5b Scrotal discomfort	5c Loss of testicular sensation	5d Urgent surgical relief of torsion and orchidoplexy of both testes

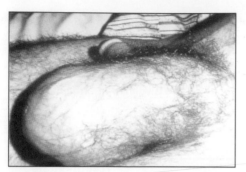

fig 4.7a

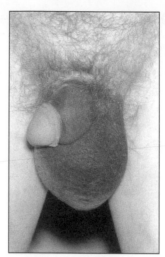

fig 4.7b

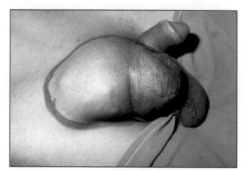

fig 4.7c

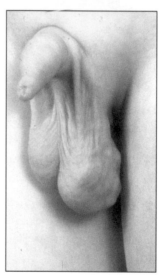

fig 4.7d

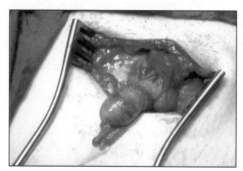

fig 4.7e

OSCE Stations

A Label each illustration with the appropriate diagnosis.

1 Testicular torsion   Fig

2 Varicocele   Fig

3 Haematocoele   Fig

4 Testicular tumour   Fig

5 Vaginal hydrocoele   Fig

4 Identify the appropriate clinical presentation and treatment for each condition in Table 4.7 by rearranging the columns in your answer.

Clinical condition history (diagnosis)	Symptoms	Signs	Treatment
1 Testicuar torsion			
2 Varicocele			
3 Haematocoele			
4 Testicular tumour			
5 Vaginal hydrocoele			

STATION 4.8

Examination

You are a medical student attached to a general medical firm. The SpR has asked you to examine a patient who is waiting to transfer to the local renal unit for their dialysis. They were admitted last night with rigors and fever which has settled with intravenous antibiotics. Please make a comprehensive assessment – including full abdominal examination. The SpR will ask you questions on completion of your examination.

(10 minute station)

STATION 4.9

Investigation

The following haematology results were obtained from patients in the renal outpatient department. Please indicate whether the following statements are **True** or **False**

(5 minute station)

Patient	Symptoms	Blood results
(A) A 21-year-old woman	Haematuria and recurrent UTIs	FBC: Hb 17.6, Hct 0.57, WCC 9.2, platelets 398
(B) A 55-year-old man	Longstanding hypertension and diabetes mellitus	FBC: Hb 6.9, MCV 82, MCH 32, WCC 6.4 platelets 288
(C) A 61-year-old man	Painless haematuria	FBC: Hb 8.1, MCV 70, WCC 13.9, platelets 539
(D) A 52-year-old woman	Bony pain	Blood film – plasma cells, ESR 132

	True	False
1 Patient (A) has polycythaemia	☐	☐
2 Patient (A) may have adult polycystic kidney disease	☐	☐
3 Patient (A) will have a low plasma erythropoetin level	☐	☐
4 Patient (B) has a hyperchromic, macrocytic anaemia	☐	☐
5 Patient (B) probably has a chronic renal disorder	☐	☐
6 Patient (B) will have a low plasma ferritin	☐	☐
7 Patient (C) has a microcytic anaemia	☐	☐
8 Patient (C) has results most consistent with a renal abscess	☐	☐
9 The results of patient (C) are consistent with active bleeding	☐	☐
10 Patient (D) should have urine sent for Bence-Jones proteins	☐	☐
11 Patient (D) would be expected to have hypocalcaemia	☐	☐
12 Patient (D) may have systemic lupus erythematosus	☐	☐

OSCE Stations

STATION 4.10

Investigation

The following biochemistry results were obtained from patients on a general medical ward. Please indicate whether the subsequent statements are **True** or **False**.

(5 minute station)

Biochemistry results

(A) U+Es – Na$^+$ 149,   K$^+$ 4.2,   HCO$_3^-$ 22,   urea 23.2,   creatinine 202, glucose 8.6

(B) U+Es – Na$^+$ 121,   K$^+$ 2.6,   HCO$_3^-$ 18,   urea 1.6,   creatinine 34,   glucose 40

(C) U+Es – Na$^+$136,   K$^+$ 4.3,   HCO$_3^-$ 15,   urea 33.6,   creatinine 563, glucose 21.1, HbA$_1$c 13.9%

(D) U+Es – Na$^+$ 127,   K$^+$ 7.2,   HCO$_3^-$ 21,   urea 22.1,   creatinine 687, CCa^{2+} 2.4

(E) U+Es – Na$^+$ 131,   K$^+$ 6.4,   HCO$_3^-$ 20,   urea 19.5,   creatinine 512, PSA 109

	True	False
1 The results of patient (A) are consistent with an obstructive nephropathy	☐	☐
2 Patient (A) may have had an acute GI bleed	☐	☐
3 Patient (B) is dehydrated	☐	☐
4 Patient (B) has diabetic nephropathy	☐	☐
5 Patient (C) has results consistent with chronic renal failure	☐	☐
6 Patient (C) may have the Kimmelstiel–Wilson lesion	☐	☐
7 Patient (D) will probably require treatment with dialysis	☐	☐
8 Patient (D) has results suggestive of multiple myeloma	☐	☐
9 Patient (E) has prerenal failure	☐	☐
10 Patient (E) should have a bone scan as part of his management	☐	☐

STATION 4.11

Investigation

The following urine samples have been reported in the microbiology laboratory. Please match the histories with the specimens below

(5 minute station)

Patient history	Urine specimen
1 A 29-year-old Asian woman with night sweats and rigors	(A) MSU – *E. coli* >10^5, WCC 750, Resistant – amoxcyllin, trimethoprim Sensitive – gentamicin, nalidixic acid
2 A 74-year-old man with an indwelling catheter	(B) EMU – AAFBs grown after six weeks
3 A 25-year-old man with a history of renal stone and acute severe loin pains	(C) Urgent microscopy – no organisms, WCC 100, red cell casts identified
4 A 33-year-old man with deranged U+Es and ankle oedema	(D) MSU – no organisms seen, WCC >1000
5 A 25-year-old pregnant woman	(E) CSU – Pseudomonas >10^5, WCC <1 Sensitive – gentamicin, ciprofloxacin

Answers

Urine specimen	Patient
(A)	
(B)	
(C)	
(D)	
(E)	

OSCE Stations

STATION 4.12

Investigation

Please match the brief patient history with the diagnosis and the correct immune marker.

(5 minute station)

Patient history	Diagnosis	Immune marker
1 A 23-year-old woman with a malar rash and features of a nephrotic syndrome	(A) Systemic sclerosis	(a) HBV
2 A 61-year-old man with severe hypertension and micro-aneurysms on renal angiography	(B) Goodpasture's disease	(b) Anti-ds DNA antigens
3 A 51-year-old woman with dysphagia, telangiectasia and calcinosis	(C) Wegener's granulomatosis	(c) aGBM antibodies
4 A 29-year-old man with a three-week history of 'flu, now presenting with a nephrotic syndrome and haemoptysis	(D) Polyarteritis nodosa	(d) cANCA
5 A 38-year-old man with a dry cough, nasal discharge and haematuria	(E) Systemic lupus erythematosus	(e) Anti-Scl 70 antibody

Answers

1 (   ) (   )
2 (   ) (   )
3 (   ) (   )
4 (   ) (   )
5 (   ) (   )

STATION 4.13

Investigation

Please indicate whether the following statements are **True** of **False**.

(5 minute station)

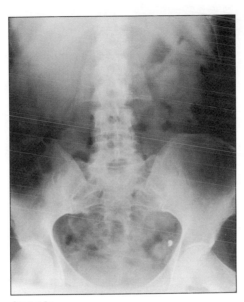

fig 4.13a

1 (fig 4.13a)	True	False
(a) This is a supine AXR	☐	☐
(b) There is a right renal stone	☐	☐
(c) The kidneys are enlarged	☐	☐
(d) There is renal calcification	☐	☐
(e) The bones are osteopaenic	☐	☐

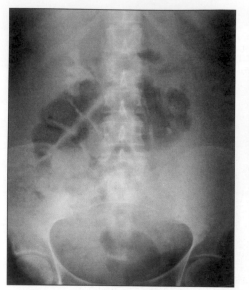

fig 4.13b

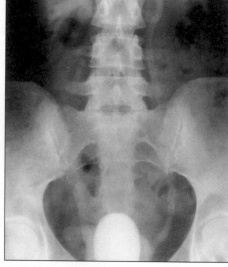

fig 4.13c

2 (fig 4.13b)	True	False
(a) Both renal outlines are visible	☐	☐
(b) There is left-sided renal calcification	☐	☐
(c) There is bladder calcification	☐	☐
(d) The bowel gas pattern is within normal limits	☐	☐
(e) The appearance of the right kidney is associated with proteus infection	☐	☐

3 (fig 4.13c)	True	False
(a) This is an IVU	☐	☐
(b) There is a wedge fracture of L3	☐	☐
(c) There is poor excretion of contrast on the left	☐	☐
(d) The sacroiliac joints are normal	☐	☐
(e) There is a foreign body in the bladder	☐	☐

STATION 4.14

Investigation

fig 4.14 is a plain radiograph of a 49-year-old man who complained of longstanding back ache, previously diagnosed and treated as musculoskeletal pain.

(5 minute station)

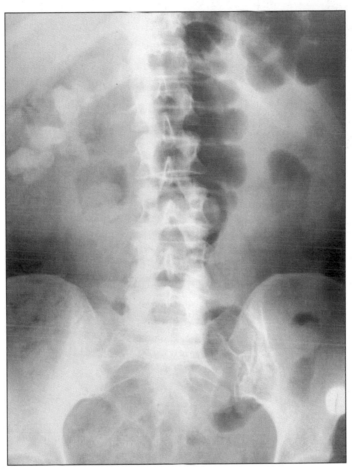

fig 4.14

1 State the abnormal finding(s).

2 List the complications of this condition.

3 How would you treat this condition?

STATION 4.15

Investigation

This is a plain radiograph of an 18-year-old Asian youth with a history of recurrent urinary tract infection.

(5 minute station)

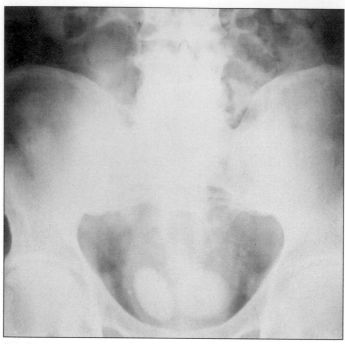

fig 4.15

1 State your diagnosis.

2 List two aetiological factors that predispose to this condition.

3 How would you treat this condition?

STATION 4.16

Investigation

fig 4.16 is a radiograph of a 38-year-old woman complaining of left-sided loin pain radiating to the groin.

(5 minute station)

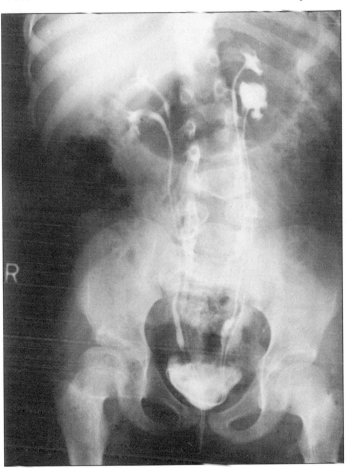

fig 4.16

1 Name the investigation.

2 State the abnormality.

3 Give another means of demonstrating this abnormality.

4 State the likely cause of this lady's symptoms.

STATION 4.17

Investigation

A 28-year-old man complained of intermittent right loin pain for five months. He underwent a radiological investigation (fig 4.17).

(5 minute station)

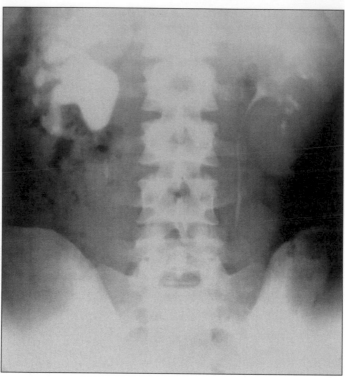

fig 4.17

1 Please name the investigation.

2 Comment on the positive findings and state your diagnosis.

3 How would you treat this condition?

4 What would be the sequelae of this lesion, left untreated?

STATION 4.18

Investigation

Please answer the questions below regarding the three investigations shown.

(5 minute station)

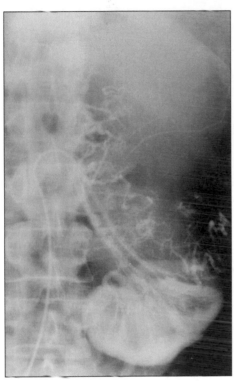

fig 4.18a

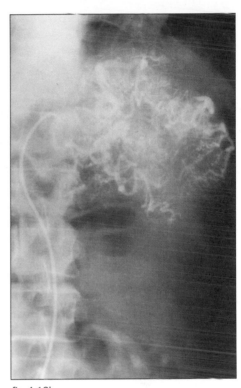

fig 4.18b

1 (figs 4.18a and 4.18b)

(a) What is this investigation?

(b) List three indications for it

(c) List two important questions you should ask the patient prior to starting the investigation.

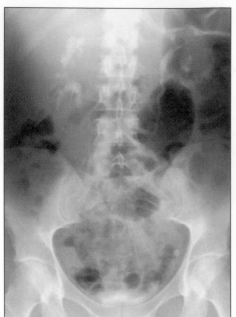

fig 4.18c

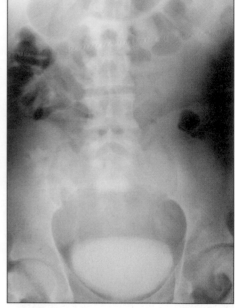

fig 4.18d

2 (fig 4.18c)

(a) What is this investigation?

(b) What is the abnormality?

(c) List three causes of this abnormality.

3 (fig 4.18d)

(a) What is this investigation?

(b) What are the abnormalities?

(c) What is the likeliest explanation?

STATION 4.19

Investigation

Shown below are five different IVU films figs 4.19a–e. (fig 4.19a is a normal IVU for comparison). Using the table, please indicate the abnormalities shown and whether they are unilateral (and the side) or bilateral. In each case you should try to give one cause or diagnosis for the abnormality.

(5 minute station)

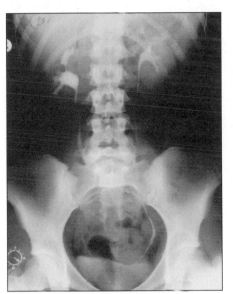

fig 4.19a

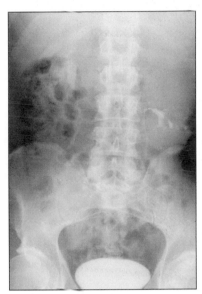

fig 4.19b

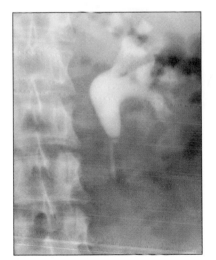

fig 4.19c

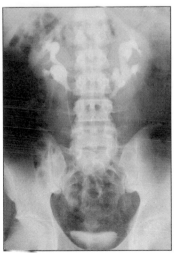

fig 4.19d

IVU	Unilateral abnormality right/left	Bilateral abnormality	Description of abnormality	Cause or diagnosis
4.19b				
4.19c				
4.19d				
4.19e				

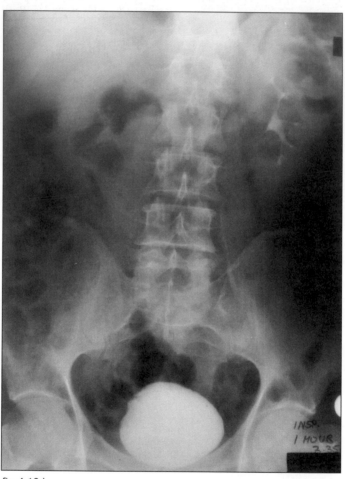

fig 4.19d

STATION 4.20

Investigation

Please label this CT scan of the abdomen and the pelvis shown below.

(5 minute station)

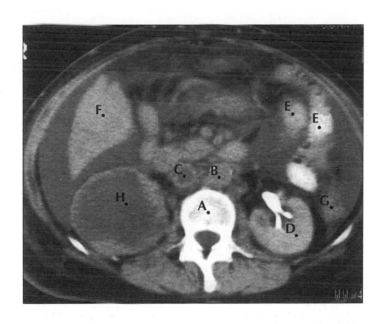

Answers

(A)   (E)

(B)   (F)

(C)   (G)

(D)   (H)

STATION 4.21

Investigation

fig 4.21a shows the normal recording obtained from an investigation of the urinary tract.

(5 minute station)

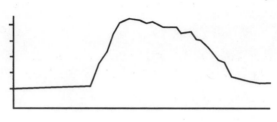

fig 4.21a

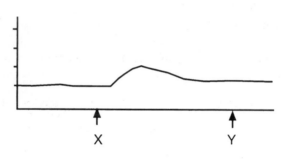

fig 4.21b

1 Name the investigation.

2 List three pathological states requiring this investigation.

3 Please label the axes in figs 4.21a and 4.21b.

4 In fig 4.21b state what happens at points x and y.

STATION 4.22

Theraputics

You will need a copy of *British National Formulary* (*BNF*) to answer this station. You are the house officer in general medical outpatients. The next patient is a 69-year-old NIDDM with known IHD and mild renal impairment. She tells you that she has been non-specifically unwell recently with nausea, dizziness on standing, and a cough.

(10 minute station)

U+Es – 2 months ago: Na$^+$ 132, K$^+$ 4.5, HCO3$^-$ 20, Ur 11.7, Cr 245
U+Es – yesterday: Na$^+$ 127, K$^+$ 3.1,   HCO3$^-$ 18, Ur 23.2, Cr 468

Medications	
	Gliclazide 160 mg bd
	Acarbose 50 mg bd
	Enalapril 10 mg bd
	Diclofenac 50 mg tds
	Aspirin 150 mg bd
	Bumetanide 3 mg od
	Omeprazole 20 mg nocte
	Amoxycillin 500 mg tds (started by her GP five days ago)
	GTN spray 1–2 puffs prn

Using the *BNF* provided and your own knowledge, answer the following questions:

1 Which of the medications could be worsening her renal function?

2 List two drugs that may affect her diabetic control.

3 List three of her drugs that may directly be causing the nausea.

4 List four drugs that may be contributing to her dizziness on standing.

5 List five investigations that you would request after her admission.

STATION 4.23

Therapeutics

The medications listed below are all used in renal tract disease. Please match the medication with the correct patient history and the relevant biochemical information.

(5 minute station)

Patient history	Drug action	Medication
1 A 73-year-old man with BPH	(A) ACE inhibitor	(a) Epoetin alpha
2 A 29-year-old woman with CRF and a normochromic, normocytic anaemia	(B) Antiandrogen	(b) Allopurinol
3 A 69-year-old man with prostatic carcinoma	(C) Anticholinergic	(c) Finasteride
4 An 81-year-old woman with urinary incontinence. Post-micturition residual <100 ml	(D) 5a reductase inhibitor	(d) Quinapril
5 A 32-year-old man with IDDM and diabetic nephropathy	(E) Xanthine oxidase inhibitor	(e) Cyproterone
6 A 55-year-old man with lymphoma and hyperuricaemia	(F) Replacement for human erythropoietin	(f) Oxybutinin

Answers

A (   ) (   )
B (   ) (   )
C (   ) (   )
D (   ) (   )
E (   ) (   )
F (   ) (   )

STATION 4.24

Procedure

Please catheterise this patient (manikin) who is in urinary retention.

(5 minute station)

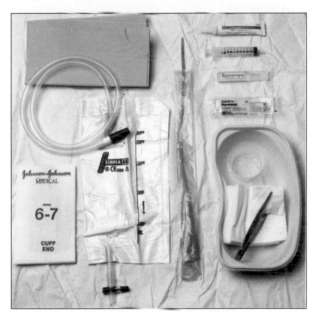

fig 4.24

Equipment provided (fig 4.24): catheterisation model, catheter trolley containing antiseptic cleansing fluid, steriledrapes, Foley size 12 urethral catheter, lubricant, forceps, catheter bag with tubing, sterile gloves, 10 ml syringe with 10 ml ampoule of normal saline.

OSCE Stations

STATION 4.25

Procedure

fig 4.25 shows a sterile appliance pack laid out for a surgical procedure.

(5 minute Station)

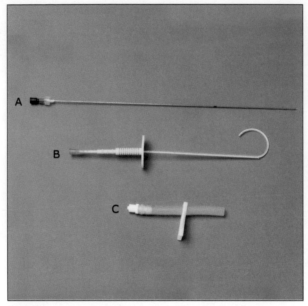

fig 4.25

1 Name items A, B and C.

2 Name the procedure the appliance is used for.

3 State the clinical diagnosis that requires this procedure.

4 Name an important clinical prerequisite prior to performing this procedure.

STATION 4.26

History/consent

A married couple attends the urology clinic with a request for a vasectomy. In order to complete the consent form for the procedure, take a relevant history from the couple.

(5 minute station)

Chapter 1:
Gastroenterology Answers

Chapter 1

Gastroenterology Answers

STATION 1.1

Patient history

I am a 24-year-old engineering student who is normally fit and well. I have been revising hard for my final exams and have been very stressed. During the last three weeks I have had bloody diarrhoea. My bowels are open once or twice an hour and I am passing semiformed/loose stools with blood and mucus, mixed and separate to the stools. I have lost 5 kg in weight and have been too tired to play squash, which I normally do twice a week. I have tried eating normally but have felt too unwell most of the time to manage anything. There seems to be no relationship between my dietary intake and the diarrhoea.

In the last week I have developed red, painful lesions on my shins, and have been feverish. I have had no recent foreign travel and no-one in my family has ever had anything similar. I have no risk factors for 'food poisoning'. I am not on any medication and do not drink alcohol. I smoke ten cigarettes per day. No-one in my family has bowel disease. I am really worried about what might be wrong and about my exams. I do not feel well enough to go out.

Assessment	Good	Adequate	Poor/not done
1 Appropriate introduction (full name and role)	☐	☐	☐
2 Explains purpose of interview	☐	☐	☐
3 Establishes duration of the illness	☐	☐	☐
4 Establishes the normal bowel habit of the patient	☐	☐	☐
5 Establishes what the patient means by diarrhoea, ie frequency and volume of stool	☐	☐	☐
6 Establishes how often the patient is opening their bowel in a 24 h period	☐	☐	☐
7 Establishes the consistency of the motion	☐	☐	☐

8　Establishes the presence of blood and
　　mucus in the stool　☐　☐　☐

9　Establishes/excludes weight loss　☐　☐　☐

10　Establishes associated gastrointestinal
　　symptoms – vomiting and abdominal pain　☐　☐　☐

11　Asks about systemic features　☐　☐　☐

12　Establishes any other risk factors for
　　diarrhoea, eg foreign travel/recent
　　contacts　☐　☐　☐

13　Establishes/excludes family history of
　　bowel disease　☐　☐　☐

14　Elicits patient's concerns and responds
　　sensitively　☐　☐　☐

15　Uses an appropriate questioning technique　☐　☐　☐

16　Avoids or explains jargon　☐　☐　☐

17　Summarises history back to the patient,
　　including concerns　☐　☐　☐

18　Systematic, organised approach　☐　☐　☐

19　Makes a reasonable attempt at the
　　diagnosis　☐　☐　☐

Diagnosis

Inflammatory bowel disease.

STATION 1.2

Patient history

I have just returned from a two month trekking holiday in Nepal. I am normally fit and well and have never had any bowel problems before. In the last 10 days I have had bloody, watery diarrhoea, with urgency. I am opening my bowels every 2–3 hours, and immediately after eating or drinking anything. I have had no vomiting, but have had intense cramping abdominal pains, particularly after food. In this period I have had a couple of episodes of fever and chills. I think I may have picked up a bug after a village feast I attended. I am not very keen on any investigations but would take medication if it was necessary.

A couple of other people on the trek were similarly unwell with fever and diarrhoea but my husband has been well. I am on no medications other than HRT after a premature menopause and drink no alcohol. I do not smoke.

I work as a librarian and these problems are really affecting my work. They are embarrassing too.

Assessment	Good	Adequate	Poor/not done
1 Appropriate introduction (full name and role)	☐	☐	☐
2 Establishes reason for patient's visit	☐	☐	☐
3 Establishes duration of present illness and excludes similar episodes	☐	☐	☐
4 Establishes where the patient went on holiday and contact history	☐	☐	☐
5 Establishes how often the patient is opening their bowels	☐	☐	☐
6 Establishes the consistency of the stool	☐	☐	☐
7 Establishes the presence of blood in the stool	☐	☐	☐
8 Asks about the presence of mucus in the stool	☐	☐	☐
9 Establishes associated features, ie pain, vomiting, fever	☐	☐	☐
10 Establishes/excludes weight loss	☐	☐	☐

11	Asks about the likely source of the infection – water, dairy products, shell fish, meat	☐ ☐ ☐
12	Elicits patient's concerns and responds sensitively	☐ ☐ ☐
13	Uses an appropriate questioning technique	☐ ☐ ☐
14	Summarises history back to the patient, including concerns	☐ ☐ ☐
15	Explains the diagnosis to the patient	☐ ☐ ☐
16	Explains the need for blood tests, stool culture and possible sigmoidoscopy and biopsy	☐ ☐ ☐
17	Gives clear, jargon-free explanation	☐ ☐ ☐
18	Checks patient's understanding of information	☐ ☐ ☐
19	Invites questions and addresses any concerns the patient may have	☐ ☐ ☐
20	Systematic, organised approach	☐ ☐ ☐

Diagnosis

Infective diarrhoea. Among other organisms amoebiasis and giardiasis should be excluded in this case.

STATION 1.3

Patient history

I am a 24-year-old legal secretary, who was previously fit and well with a normal bowel habit until four months ago. Since then I have been passing offensive, pale, porridge-like stools up to eight to ten times per day. The stools float and are difficult to flush away.

During my illness I have lost 10 kg in weight, have lost my appetite and feel extremely tired, to the point where I am now missing a lot of time from work. I have no abdominal pain, nausea or vomiting and have not passed any blood or mucus rectally. I have had no fever or systemic upset. I am really concerned about the weight loss – doesn't this mean that it could be something serious?

I have never been abroad and have had no recent contacts with anyone with similar symptoms. There is no family history of bowel problems. I drink 5–10 units of alcohol per week (mainly white wine) and smoke 20 cigarettes per day. I am on no medications other than the OCP.

Assessment	Good	Adequate	Poor/not done
1 Appropriate introduction (full name and role)	☐	☐	☐
2 Explains purpose of interview	☐	☐	☐
3 Establishes the duration and nature of the presenting complaint	☐	☐	☐
4 Establishes the normal bowel habit of the patient	☐	☐	☐
5 Establishes the frequency and volume of diarrhoea	☐	☐	☐
6 Establishes stools have the characteristics of steatorrhoea	☐	☐	☐
7 Establishes/excludes the presence of blood and mucous PR	☐	☐	☐
8 Establishes the associated features of anorexia, weight loss and lethargy	☐	☐	☐
9 Establishes/excludes recent foreign travel or contacts	☐	☐	☐

Answers

10 Establishes/excludes family history of
  bowel disease ☐ ☐ ☐

11 Elicits patient's concerns and responds
  sensitively ☐ ☐ ☐

12 Uses an appropriate questioning
  technique ☐ ☐ ☐

13 Avoids or explains jargon ☐ ☐ ☐

14 Summarises history back to the patient,
  including concerns ☐ ☐ ☐

15 Establishes the diagnosis of malabsorption
  and makes a reasonable attempt at
  the differential diagnosis ☐ ☐ ☐

16 Systematic approach ☐ ☐ ☐

SP to mark

17 The student was empathic ☐ ☐ ☐

Diagnosis

Malabsorption secondary to coeliac disease.

Comment

Differential diagnosis:

- Coeliac disease and dermatitis herpetiformis
- Infective – tropical sprue, bacterial overgrowth, Whipple's disease
- Giardia, cryptosporidium
- Small bowel lymphoma
- Pancreatic insufficiency
- Small bowel resection – short bowel syndrome, blind loop syndrome
- Iatrogenic – radiation enteritis, drugs, eg cholestyramine

STATION 1.4

Patient history

I am a 36-year-old chronic alcohol abuser with repeated admissions with upper GI bleeds secondary to oesophageal varices. I have had an endonscopy, and on two or three occasions the varices have been injected. I have been out on a large alcoholic binge and started vomiting fresh blood about an hour ago. I have vomited twice, each time bringing up about a cup or two of blood. I have some retrosternal and epigastric pain and feel nauseated. I have not had any melaena or blood PR. I do not take any NSAIDs and do not have any other risk factors for GI bleeding. I am healthy apart from the varices but I do smoke moderately.

Assessment	Good	Adequate	Poor/not done
1 Appropriate introduction (full name and role)	☐	☐	☐
2 Explains purpose of interview	☐	☐	☐
3 Establishes the nature of the haematemesis, ie fresh blood or coffee grounds	☐	☐	☐
4 Establishes the present number of haemetemeses and the volume of each haematemesis	☐	☐	☐
5 Establishes the absence of melaena stool and fresh blood PR	☐	☐	☐
6 Establishes previous episodes of haematemesis and hospital admissions	☐	☐	☐
7 Asks about associated symptoms, eg epigastric pain recent weight loss, anorexia, dyspepsia	☐	☐	☐

Answers

8 Establishes or excludes the risk factors
   for upper GI bleed:

   Use of NSAIDs   ☐   ☐

   Alcohol excess   ☐   ☐

   Previous peptic ulcer disease   ☐   ☐

   Known oesophageal varices   ☐   ☐

   Medications – eg warfarin   ☐   ☐

9 Uses an appropriate questioning
   technique   ☐   ☐   ☐

10 Avoids or explains jargon   ☐   ☐   ☐

11 Makes a reasonable attempt at the
   diagnosis   ☐   ☐   ☐

12 Systematic and organised approach ☐   ☐   ☐

SP to mark

13 The student was non-judgemental   ☐   ☐   ☐

Diagnosis

Alcohol-related chronic liver disease with known oesophageal varices.

STATION 1.5

Patient history

I am a 32-year-old stockbroker, and am normally fit and well. Like all stockbrokers I suppose I drink and smoke too much and live on takeaways. (When pressed admits to the exact amounts – I smoke 30 cigarettes per day, drink 30–40 units of alcohol per week in the form of lager and spirits.)

In the past six months I have had increasing upper abdominal pain, this is particularly bad when I am under stress or have been on a bit of a binge. The pain is burning in nature and radiates through to my back and occasionally behind my breast bone. It is relieved with Rennies and Alka-Seltzers. It is usually worse when I am hungry and better with meals. It makes me feel rather irritable and I'm concerned that it is more than just indigestion.

I have been otherwise well, with no other GI symptoms. My weight is stable and my appetite is fine. I have never vomited up blood but I did have some black stools one morning after a particularly bad episode a few weeks ago. I do not take any pain killers and have never had any peptic ulcers, hiatus hernias or gastritis in the past. I have had no symptoms suggestive of anaemia, eg shortness of breath, chest pain or faints, but have been feeling tired of late.

Assessment	Good	Adequate	Poor/not done
1 Appropriate introduction (full name and role)	☐	☐	☐
2 Explains purpose of interview	☐	☐	☐
3 Establishes onset of symptoms	☐	☐	☐
4 Establishes characteristics of the abdominal pain:			
Site and radiation	☐	☐	☐
Exacerbating factors	☐	☐	☐
Relieving factors	☐	☐	☐
5 Establishes/excludes haematemesis, melaena or fresh blood PR	☐	☐	☐
6 Establishes/excludes dyspepsia, retrosternal burning and water brash	☐	☐	☐

7 Establishes associated GI symptoms, eg weight loss, anorexia, nausea and vomiting ☐ ☐ ☐

8 Establishes risk factors for peptic ulcer disease and upper GI inflammation:

Use of pain killers ☐ ☐ ☐

Alcohol excess ☐ ☐ ☐

Smoker ☐ ☐ ☐

Previous ulcer ☐ ☐ ☐

Known hiatus hernia ☐ ☐ ☐

GI inflammation, eg gastritis ☐ ☐ ☐

9 Establishes/excludes symptoms of anaemia ☐ ☐ ☐

10 Elicits patient's concerns and responds sensitively ☐ ☐ ☐

11 Uses an appropriate questioning technique ☐ ☐ ☐

12 Avoids or explains jargon ☐ ☐ ☐

13 Summarises history back to the patient, including concerns ☐ ☐ ☐

14 Makes a reasonable attempt at the diagnosis ☐ ☐ ☐

15 Systematic, organised approach ☐ ☐ ☐

Diagnosis

Peptic ulcer disease.

STATION 1.6

1 **True** – this allows not only direct visual evidence of the cause but also the taking of biopsies and performance of a CLO test.

2 **False** – an iron deficiency anaemia is associated with a low plasma ferritin.

3 **True** – this is usually associated with chronic cases of iron deficiency.

4 **False** – a microcytic anaemia produces a low MCV.

5 **True** – CLO:campylocbacter-like organism = *Helicobacter pylori*.

6 **True** – triple therapy is used in ulcer healing and eradication of *Helicobacter pylori*.

7 **False** – it is usually given for 1 week.

8 **True** – clarithromycin is given with amoxycillin and a proton pump inhibitor.

9 **False** – cimetidine is an H_2 antagonist.

10 **False** – he may require 3–6 months of treatment but provided he stops smoking and reduces his alcohol intake, he should avoid recurrence. Maintenance or long-term therapy with a proton pump inhibitor is only occasionally required.

STATION 1.7

Patient history

I am a 47-year-old carpet salesman with a long history of peptic ulcer disease and gastro-oesophageal reflux. I have a six month history of intermittent difficulty in swallowing solids. I can manage most foods most of the time but occasionally foods, like bread and potatoes, seem to stick 'behind the lower part of my breast bone'. I have lost a little weight, about 2 to 3 kg, but have had no other associated gastrointestinal symptoms.

I am generally well and have had no major illness or admissions to hospital in the past. I am a non-smoker and drink 5–10 units of alcohol per week, principally in the form of red wine. I am worried that I have cancer because I have heard in the papers that this can be a symptom.

Assessment	Good	Adequate	Poor/not done
1 Appropriate introduction (full name and role)	☐	☐	☐
2 Establishes reason for patient's visit	☐	☐	☐
3 Establishes the duration and nature of the presenting illness	☐	☐	☐
4 Establishes the level of the dysphagia, ie pharynx, upper, mid or lower oesophagus	☐	☐	☐
5 Establishes the degree of dysphagia, ie solids/liquids	☐	☐	☐
6 Establishes the rate and nature of progression	☐	☐	☐
7 Establishes/excludes presence of regurgitation	☐	☐	☐
8 Establishes history of peptic ulcer disease and reflux	☐	☐	☐
9 Establishes/excludes symptoms of GI bleeding – melaena, haematemesis, blood PR	☐	☐	☐
10 Establishes/excludes associated gastrointestinal features eg abdominal pain, nausea and vomiting, weight loss	☐	☐	☐

11 Excludes risk factors for oesophageal
carcinoma ☐ ☐ ☐

12 Establishes any associated features of
systemic diseases or relevant previous
medical history ☐ ☐ ☐

13 Elicits patient's concerns and responds
sensitively ☐ ☐ ☐

14 Uses an appropriate questioning technique ☐ ☐ ☐

15 Avoids or explains jargon ☐ ☐ ☐

16 Summarises history back to the patient,
including concerns ☐ ☐ ☐

17 Makes a reasonable attempt at the
diagnosis ☐ ☐ ☐

18 Systematic, organised approach ☐ ☐ ☐

SP to mark

19 The doctor was empathic ☐ ☐ ☐

Diagnosis

Benign stricture secondary to long-term gastro-oesophageal reflux disease (GORD).

STATION 1.8

Patient history

I am 33 years old and I have been unwell for about two months. Initially I thought I just had a touch of 'flu with a slight fever and aching joints and muscles. However, in the last week or so I have developed yellow skin and eyes. I feel very lethargic and generally unwell.

In response to questioning only

I drink 20 to 30 pints of beer per week and an occasional whisky. In the past I have been an intravenous drug abuser and shared needles on occasions. Currently I am off drugs. A recent HIV test I had was negative.

I have not travelled abroad and have had no sexual contacts with prostitutes. I have had no homosexual contacts, no blood transfusions and no regular medications. I remember my mother saying I was born jaundiced but I have never had any further episodes. I have no other gastric symptoms although I have lost 4 kg in the past six months. My stools and urine are normal in colour and consistency. I am working in a sorting depot of a large Post Office and smoke 10 to 20 cigarettes per day. I do not really feel up to work and I'm not able to do much with my children.

Assessment	Good	Adequate	Poor/not done
1 Appropriate introduction (full name and role)	☐	☐	☐
2 Explains purpose of interview and gains consent	☐	☐	☐
3 Establishes reason for coming to the Emergency Department	☐	☐	☐
4 Establishes the duration and nature of the presenting symptoms	☐	☐	☐
5 Establishes previous episodes of jaundice and cause	☐	☐	☐

6 Establishes risk/symptoms of infective
   hepatitis:

   Prodromal symptoms/fever   ☐   ☐

   Foreign travel   ☐   ☐

   Sexual contacts   ☐   ☐

   Recent contacts   ☐   ☐

   Intravenous drug abuse   ☐   ☐

   Previous transfusions   ☐   ☐

7 Establishes alcohol consumption and
   duration   ☐   ☐   ☐

8 Establishes colour and consistency of
   stools and urine   ☐   ☐   ☐

9 Establishes medications

10 Establishes systemic symptoms –
   weight loss, abdominal pain, diarrhoea,
   steatorrhoea   ☐   ☐   ☐

11 Elicits patient's concerns and responds
   sensitively   ☐   ☐   ☐

12 Uses an appropriate questioning
   technique   ☐   ☐   ☐

13 Avoids or explains jargon   ☐   ☐   ☐

14 Summarises history back to the patient,
   including concerns   ☐   ☐   ☐

15 Makes a reasonable attempt at the
   diagnosis   ☐   ☐   ☐

16 Systematic, organised approach   ☐   ☐   ☐

SP to mark

17 The student was non-judgemental   ☐   ☐   ☐

Diagnosis

This patient has risk factors for viral hepatitis complicated by possible alcoholic liver disease. He will need investigation to exclude viral causes including liver biopsy. He should be counselled about alcohol consumption.

STATION 1.9

Patient history

Three months ago I noticed dark blood mixed in the motions, which are hard but occasionally very loose with slime. My appetite is poor, I have lost a little weight and I am not eating well, as I feel bloated with crampy pains in the abdomen following meals. I had a severe attack of bowel cramps a few years ago. I had an X-ray of the bowels which showed I had diverticulitis. I was placed on a course of tablets but have been constipated most of my life. I had my gall bladder removed for stones many years ago and am on water and blood pressure tablets. I live alone and I manage very well. I don't drink or smoke. I am concerned that I have cancer because I have symptoms that I have read about in magazines. I don't want to tell my daughters because they will make a fuss.

Assessment	Good	Adequate	Poor/not done
1 Appropriate introduction (full name and role)	☐	☐	☐
2 Explains purpose of interview	☐	☐	☐
3 Establishes presenting complaint:			
Passage of blood/slime/melaena	☐	☐	☐
Constipation alternating with diarrhoea	☐	☐	☐
Tenesmus, pruritus, piles	☐	☐	☐
4 Asks about poor appetite/weight loss	☐	☐	☐
5 Asks about abdominal cramps and bloating	☐	☐	☐
6 Establishes past history of bowel problems and outcome	☐	☐	☐
7 Establishes current dietary habits and lifestyle	☐	☐	☐
8 Elicits patient's concerns and responds sensitively	☐	☐	☐
9 Uses an appropriate questioning technique	☐	☐	☐
10 Avoids or explains jargon	☐	☐	☐

11 Summarises history back to the patient,
     including concerns   ☐   ☐   ☐

12 Makes a reasonable attempt at the
     diagnosis   ☐   ☐   ☐

13 Systematic, organised approach   ☐   ☐   ☐

SP to mark

14 It was easy for me to talk to this student ☐   ☐   ☐

Diagnosis

Inflammatory bowel disease.

Comment

A long history of episodic diarrhoea with malaise and the passage of mucus is
indicative of inflammatory bowel disease, although less severe symptoms may
suggest an irritable bowel syndrome. Abdominal bloating and cramps point to
subacute colonic obstruction, usually from a constricting tumour. This is a late
presentation in tumours of the distal colon but may be the only symptom in tumours
of the proximal colon. A long history of constipation and diverticular disease usually
go hand-in-hand, and rectal bleeding from a focus of diverticulitis is not uncommon.
Massive bleeding results from erosion of blood vessels at the base of a diverticulum,
and is uncommon in an ulcerating tumour.

STATION 1.10

Patient history

I have suffered from piles on and off for the past 25 years. They now come out when I go to the toilet and sometimes I have to push them back. There is usually blood on the toilet paper and occasionally splashes of blood in the toilet bowl. I had the piles injected a few years ago and use Anusol suppositories when they become troublesome. I am a long-distance lorry driver, and as I spend days on the road, my meals are not regular, and I tend to be constipated. I am generally healthy and have had no major illnesses. I am trying to get my weight down. It is quite embarrassing to talk about this problem.

Assessment	Good	Adequate	Poor/not done
1 Appropriate introduction (full name and role)	☐	☐	☐
2 Explains purpose of interview	☐	☐	☐
3 Establishes presenting complaint	☐	☐	☐
4 Establishes the duration of symptoms and treatment	☐	☐	☐
5 Establishes dietary and bowel habits: excludes passage of blood and mucus	☐	☐	☐
6 Establishes general lifestyle	☐	☐	☐
7 Uses an appropriate questioning technique	☐	☐	☐
8 Avoids or explains jargon	☐	☐	☐
9 Summarises history back to the patient, including concerns	☐	☐	☐
10 Makes a reasonable attempt at the diagnosis	☐	☐	☐
11 Systematic, organised approach	☐	☐	☐
SP to mark			
12 I felt comfortable talking to this student	☐	☐	☐

Diagnosis

Haemorrhoids.

Haemorrhoids are a common and benign ailment, affecting 10% of the population. Piles are associated with, and may indeed be precipitated by, poor dietary habit and constipation. Small piles (first degree haemorrhoids) may respond to a high residue diet alone. Large and troublesome piles that have responded poorly to sclerotherapy or rubber banding require surgery. It is important to bear in mind that piles may be a red herring in patients with rectal bleeding caused by an occult colonic tumour.

STATION 1.11

Assessment	Good	Adequate	Poor/not done
1 Appropriate introduction (full name and role)	☐	☐	☐
2 Explains purpose of examination – gains verbal consent	☐	☐	☐
3 Candidate washes their hands using the alcohol handwash provided (no marks if candidate only expresses the need to wash if handwash is provided)	☐	☐	☐
4 Ensures patient is appropriately exposed, lying comfortably and as flat as they can manage	☐	☐	☐
5 Asks patient to take a deep breath in – commenting on the presence or absence of obvious distress or masses	☐	☐	☐
6 Comments on the presence/absence of: oedema, abdominal scars, obvious masses, asymmetry of abdomen, abdominal swelling/distention, stoma bag, jaundice, anaemia, signs of chronic liver disease	☐	☐	☐

7 Returns to patient's side – examines the hands commenting on presence/absence of nail clubbing, leuconychia, koilonychia, anaemia, palmar erythema, Dupuytrens contracture ± liver flap   ☐   ☐   ☐

8 Examines the patient's face – commenting on presence/absence of jaundice, anaemia, dentition, ulceration of oral mucosa and hepatic fetor   ☐   ☐   ☐

9 Examines the patient's neck – specifically commenting on the presence/absence of left supraclavicular fossa lymphadenopathy. **Examiner asks 'What are you examining for?'** Answer – Virchow's node, Trossier's sign.   ☐   ☐   ☐

10 Examines the patient's chest – commenting on the presence/absence of spider naevi, gynaecomastia and loss of male distribution of hair   ☐   ☐   ☐

11 Ascertains if the patient has any pain in the abdomen and if it is localised to any particular area   ☐   ☐   ☐

12 Kneels or bends to an appropriate level to examine the patient's abdomen   ☐   ☐

13 Reassures patient:

'I'll be gentle as possible'   ☐   ☐

'My hands are warm'   ☐   ☐

14 Examines all areas of the abdomen in a systematic manner leaving painful areas till last   ☐   ☐   ☐

15 Examines all areas both superficially and deeply   ☐   ☐   ☐

16 Uses correct technique and observes
patient for signs of discomfort throughout ☐ ☐ ☐

17 Examines for hepatomegaly –
appropriately moving hand:

With respiration of patient ☐ ☐

*From right iliac fossa up to the right
costal margin* ☐ ☐

Using appropriate technique ☐ ☐

18 Percusses for upper and lower border
of liver ☐ ☐ ☐

19 Examines for splenomegaly – appropriately
moving hand:

With respiration of patient ☐ ☐

*From right iliac fossa up to the left
costal margin* ☐ ☐

Using appropriate technique ☐ ☐

20 Percusses for upper/lower border of
spleen ☐ ☐ ☐

21 Examines for right and left kidney –
attempting to:

Bimanually ballots the kidneys ☐ ☐

Using appropriate technique ☐ ☐

22 If appropriate, examines for ascites
correctly demonstrates 'shifting dullness' ☐ ☐ ☐

23 Palpates for inguinal lymphadenopathy ☐ ☐ ☐

24 Auscultates for bowel sounds ☐ ☐

25 Completes examination by ensuring
patient is covered and comfortable to
maintain dignity; thanks patient ☐ ☐ ☐

26 Requests:

The observations BP, pulse, temperature, urinalysis/O₂ sats ☐   ☐

To examine the external genitalia ☐   ☐

To perform a digital rectal examination (PR) ☐   ☐

27 Presents findings in a fluent, logical manner ☐   ☐   ☐

28 Presents an appropriate differential diagnosis or causes of the condition ☐   ☐   ☐

Common questions posed at the end of this station:

1   Why would you like to see the observation chart?
2   Why do you want to do a PR examination? What might you find?
3   In a patient of this age what are the likely causes of
     (a) Hepatomegaly
     (b) Splenomegaly
     (c) Hepatosplenomegaly
     (d) Renal mass(es)
     (e) Ascites?

STATION 1.12

Assessment	Good	Adequate	Poor/not done
1 Appropriate introduction (full name and role)	☐	☐	☐
2 Explains purpose of examination – obtains verbal consent	☐	☐	☐
3 Ensures patient is appropriately exposed, lying comfortably as flat as they can manage	☐	☐	☐
4 Stands at the end of the bed and observes patient; comments on the presence/absence – oedema/abdominal scars, obvious masses, asymmetry of abdomen, abdominal swelling/ distention, stoma bag, jaundice, anaemia, signs of chronic liver disease	☐	☐	☐
5 Ascertains if the patient has any pain in the abdomen and if it is localised to any particular area	☐	☐	☐
6 Kneels or bends to an appropriate level to examine the patient's abdomen		☐	☐
7 Reassures patient:			
'I'll be as gentle as possible'		☐	☐
'My hands are warm'		☐	☐
8 Examines all areas of the abdomen in a systematic manner leaving painful areas till last	☐	☐	☐
9 Examines all areas both superficially and deeply	☐	☐	☐
10 Uses correct technique and observes patient for signs of discomfort throughout	☐	☐	☐

11 Examines for hepatomegaly –
    appropriately moving hand

    With respiration of patient ☐ ☐

    *From right iliac fossa up to the right
    costal margin* ☐ ☐

    Using appropriate technique ☐ ☐

12 Percusses for upper and lower border
    of liver ☐ ☐ ☐

13 Examines for splenomegaly – appropriately
    moving hand:

    With respiration of patient ☐ ☐

    *From right iliac fossa up to the left costal
    margin* ☐ ☐

    Using appropriate technique ☐ ☐

14 Percusses for upper/lower border of
    spleen ☐ ☐ ☐

15 Examines for right and left kidney –
    attempting to:

    Bimanually ballot the kidneys ☐ ☐

    Using appropriate technique ☐ ☐

16 If appropriate, examines for ascites,
    correctly demonstrates 'shifting dullness' ☐ ☐ ☐

17 Palpates for inguinal lymphadenopathy ☐ ☐ ☐

18 Auscultates for bowel sounds ☐ ☐ ☐

19 Completes examination by ensuring
    patient is covered and comfortable to
    maintain dignity; thanks patient ☐ ☐ ☐

20 Requests:

    *The observations BP, pulse, Temperature,
    urinalysis/O_2 sats* ☐ ☐

    To examine the external genitalia ☐ ☐

    *To perform a digital rectal examination
    (PR)* ☐ ☐

	Good	Adequate	Poor/not done
21 Presents findings in a fluent, logical manner	☐	☐	☐
22 Presents an appropriate differential diagnosis or causes of the condition	☐	☐	☐

This is a 10 minute station and is principally used in junior clinical years to assess examination technique rather than diagnostic skills.

STATION 1.13

Assessment	Good	Adequate	Poor/not done
1 Appropriate introduction (full name and role)	☐	☐	☐
2 Explains purpose of examination – gains verbal consent	☐	☐	☐
3 Candidate washes their hands using the alcohol handwash provided (no marks if candidate only expresses the need to wash if handwash is provided)	☐	☐	☐
4 Ensures patient is appropriately exposed, lying comfortably as flat as they can manage	☐	☐	☐
5 Stands at the end of the bed and observes patient; comments on the presence/absence of:			
Oedema			
Abdominal scars	☐	☐	☐
Obvious masses	☐	☐	☐
Asymmetry of abdomen	☐	☐	☐
Abdominal swelling/distention	☐	☐	☐
Stoma bag	☐	☐	☐
Jaundice	☐	☐	☐
Anaemia	☐	☐	☐
Signs of chronic liver disease	☐	☐	☐

Examiner asks, 'What are the relevant observations?'

Answers:

Not clinically jaundiced	☐	☐	☐
No bruising/pruritis marks	☐	☐	☐
Tattoos – presence/absence	☐	☐	☐
Signs of chronic liver disease (presence/absence)	☐	☐	☐
Ascites and abdominal distention	☐	☐	☐
Abdominal masses	☐	☐	☐
Hepatosplenomegaly	☐	☐	☐

6 Returns to patient's side – examines the hands commenting on presence/absence of nail clubbing, leuconychia, koilonychia, anaemia, palmar erythema, Dupuytrens contracture ± liver flap ☐ ☐ ☐

7 Examiner asks 'comment on your relevant findings' Student describes presence/absence of:

Signs of chronic liver disease	☐	☐	☐
Anaemia and signs of iron deficiency	☐	☐	☐
BP and pulse	☐	☐	☐

8 Examines the patient's face – commenting on presence/absence of jaundice/ anaemia/dentition/oral mucosa – ulceration/hepatic fetor ☐ ☐ ☐

9 Examines the patient's neck – specifically commenting on the presence/absence of left supraclavicular fossa lymphadenopathy, Virchow's node, and Trossier's sign ☐ ☐ ☐

10 Examines the patient's chest – commenting on the presence/absence of spider naevi, gynaecomastia and loss of male distribution of hair ☐ ☐ ☐

11 Ascertains if the patient has any pain
    in the abdomen and if it is localised to
    any particular area   ☐   ☐   ☐

12 Kneels or bends to an appropriate level to
    examine the patient's abdomen   ☐   ☐   ☐

13 Reassures patient:

    'I'll be gentle and will try not to hurt you' ☐   ☐   ☐

    'My hands are warm'   ☐   ☐   ☐

14 Examines all areas of the abdomen in
    a systematic manner   ☐   ☐   ☐

15 Examines all areas both superficially
    and deeply   ☐   ☐   ☐

16 Uses correct technique and observes
    patient for signs of discomfort throughout ☐   ☐   ☐

17 Examines for hepatomegaly – moving
    hand appropriately with respiration of
    the patient   ☐   ☐   ☐

18 Percusses for upper and lower border
    of liver   ☐   ☐   ☐

19 Examines for splenomegaly – moving
    hand appropriately with respiration of
    patient   ☐   ☐   ☐

20 Percusses for upper/lower border of
    spleen   ☐   ☐   ☐

21 Examines for right and left kidney –
    attempting to ballot the kidneys   ☐   ☐   ☐

22 If appropriate, examines for ascites,
    looks for 'shifting dullness'   ☐   ☐   ☐

23 Palpates for inguinal lymphadenopathy   ☐   ☐   ☐

24 Auscultates for bowel sounds   ☐   ☐

25 Completes examination by making
    patient comfortable and ensuring they
    are covered to maintain dignity   ☐   ☐   ☐

26 Requests:

The observations BP, pulse, Temperature,
urinalysis, O_2 sats   ☐   ☐   ☐

To examine the external genitalia   ☐   ☐

To perform a digital rectal examination
(PR)   ☐   ☐

27 **Examiner asks:**

(a) 'Why would you examine the external genitalia of this male patient?'

Correct answer: 'To check for gonadal atrophy, tesicular mass.'

(b) 'Why would you do a PR examination?'

Correct answer: 'To check for stool colour (pale in steatorrhoea or obstructive jaundice). Prostatomegaly, rectal tumours, ± melaena.'

(c) 'Why may this patient be pyrexial?'

Correct answers: 'systemic infection eg legionella, mycoplasma, EBV acute viral hepatitis, gallstones, cholecystitis, cholangitis, hepatic abscess.'

28 Presents findings in a fluent,
   logical manner   ☐   ☐   ☐

29 Presents an appropriate differential
   diagnosis or causes of the condition   ☐   ☐   ☐

STATION 1.14

Assessment	Good	Adequate	Poor/not done
1 Appropriate introduction (full name and role)	☐	☐	☐
2 Explains examination to patient and carer; gains verbal consent	☐	☐	☐
3 Candidate washes their hands using the alcohol handwash provided (no marks if candidate only expresses the need to wash if handwash is provided)	☐	☐	☐
4 Checks patient is comfortable when placed supine prior to lying them down	☐	☐	☐
5 Exposes patient appropriately to observe abdomen, while trying to maintain patient dignity	☐	☐	☐
6 Observes patient from end of the bed and comments on:			
Patient in obvious distress	☐	☐	☐
Need for appropriate analgesia before continuing	☐	☐	☐
7 Observes and comments on:			
Perfusion/wellbeing of patient	☐	☐	☐
Presence/absence of:			
Jaundice and anaemia	☐	☐	☐
Abdomen – scars, masses, obvious organomegaly, fistulae	☐	☐	☐
8 Returns and kneels on the right-hand side of the patient		☐	☐
9 Reassures and calms patient about examination and technique	☐	☐	☐
10 Enquires about area of maximal tenderness – starts examination away from this site	☐	☐	☐

11 Systematically palpates the surface
of the abdomen both superficially
and deeply ☐ ☐ ☐

12 Comments on any areas of guarding
or presence of rigidity ☐ ☐ ☐

13 Attempts to elicit rebound guarding in
areas of maximal tenderness ☐ ☐ ☐

14 Comments on the presence of any
masses ☐ ☐

15 Examines (recognising the limitations of
the assessment) for:

Hepatomegaly ☐ ☐ ☐

Splenomegaly ☐ ☐ ☐

Renal enlargement ☐ ☐ ☐

Hernial orifices ☐ ☐ ☐

16 Attempts to elicit Rovsing's sign ☐ ☐ ☐

17 Auscultates for and comments on
bowel sounds ☐ ☐ ☐

18 **Examiner asks**

*'Can you show me where McBurney's
point is?'* ☐ ☐ ☐

*'Can you explain how and why you would
perform a psoas test or an obturator
test?'* ☐ ☐ ☐

19 Student completes the examination by
requesting to:

Perform a digital rectal examination ☐ ☐ ☐

*Look at the observation chart for signs of
sepsis – pyrexia, tachycardia, hypotension,
oxygenation* ☐ ☐ ☐

*Dip the urine to exclude urinary sepsis or
renal disease* ☐ ☐ ☐

20	Thanks patient and carer and covers patient maintaining comfort and dignity	☐	☐	☐
21	Presents findings in a fluent, logical manner with appropriate differential diagnosis	☐	☐	☐
22	Performs examination in a professional manner	☐	☐	☐

Comment

Acute abdominal problems are commonly simulated in OSCEs by actors. They provide a good opportunity to observe how the student deals with an acutely 'sick' patient, including how they examine them. The use of children in OSCEs is limited for obvious reasons but digital and video recordings are now being used in OSCE stations to assess students. The recordings may form the basis of a structured viva or more commonly are assessed with written or computer-based tests.

The classical findings of appendicitis are localised tenderness in the right iliac fossa which may be associated with signs of peritoneal irritation. These in turn may be associated with fever, vomiting and anorexia. However, fewer than 50% of patients present in this classical manner and many patients had a normal appendix removed before ultrasound and CT scan of the abdomen were used to confirm the diagnosis.

McBurney's point is the half-way point between the umbilicus and the right anterior superior iliac spine (Professor Charles McBurney (1845–1913) – US surgeon). The Psoas test demonstrates peritoneal irritation by causing increased abdominal pain by flexion of the right hip against resistance. A similar test, the obturator test, will increase the abdominal pain by flexing and internally rotating the right hip. Rovsing's sign is elicited by pressing in the LEFT iliac fossa which produces RIGHT iliac fossa pain (Niels Rovsing (1862–1927) – Danish surgeon; co-founder of the Danish Surgical Society). Intimate examination such as per rectal and vaginal examination of children should only be performed with parental consent and, as with any adult, a chaperone present. The older child (aged 10 years and above) may not wish to have their parent or guardian present and their wishes should be respected.

The differential diagnosis of right iliac fossa pain includes:
- Renal sepsis, stones and urinary tract infection
- Ectopic pregnancy (women of childbearing years who are sexually active)
- Ovarian cysts and torsion
- Pelvic inflammatory disease (PID)
- Caecal tumours (older people)
- Adenitis

STATION 1.15

Assessment	Good	Adequate	Poor/not done
1 Appropriate introduction (full name and role)	☐	☐	☐
2 Explains examination and gains verbal consent	☐	☐	☐
3 Checks patient is comfortable when placed supine prior to lying them down	☐	☐	☐
4 Exposes patient appropriately to observe abdomen, whilst trying to maintain dignity	☐	☐	☐
5 Observes patient from end of the bed: comments on			
Patient in obvious distress	☐	☐	☐
Need for appropriate analgesia before continuing	☐	☐	☐
6 Observes and comments on			
Perfusion/wellbeing of patient presence/absence of Jaundice and anaemia	☐	☐	☐
Abdomen – scars, masses, obvious organomegaly, fistulae	☐	☐	☐
7 Returns and kneels on the right-hand side of the patient	☐	☐	☐
8 Reassures patient about examination technique	☐	☐	☐
9 Enquires about area of maximal tenderness – starts examination away from this site	☐	☐	☐
10 Systematically palpates the surface of the abdomen both superficially and deeply	☐	☐	☐
11 Comments on any areas of guarding or prescence of rigidity	☐	☐	☐
12 Attempts to elicit rebound guarding in areas of maximal tenderness	☐	☐	☐

13 Comments on the presence of any masses ☐ ☐ ☐

14 Examines (recognising the limitations of the assessment) for

    Hepatomeqaly ☐ ☐ ☐

    Splenomegaly ☐ ☐ ☐

    Renal enlargement ☐ ☐ ☐

    Hernial orifices ☐ ☐ ☐

15 Auscultates for and comments on bowel sounds ☐ ☐ ☐

16 Student completes the examination by requesting to

    Perform a digital rectal examination ☐ ☐ ☐

    Looks at the observation chart for signs of sepsis – pyrexia, tachycardia, hypotension, oxygenation ☐ ☐ ☐

    Dip the urine to exclude urinary sepsis or renal disease ☐ ☐ ☐

17 Thanks patient and covers patient maintaining comfort and dignity ☐ ☐ ☐

18 Presents findings in a fluent, logical manner with appropriate differential diagnosis ☐ ☐ ☐

19 **Examiner asks**

    What investigations would you arrange? ☐ ☐ ☐

    How would you manage this patient? ☐ ☐ ☐
    (see below)

20 Performs examination in a professional manner ☐ ☐ ☐

Answers

Comment

The usual cause of peritoneal irritation or a mass in the left lower quadrant in an older patient is acute diverticulitis or diverticular mass of the sigmoid colon. The differential diagnosis includes

- ureteric and renal colic; renal tract sepsis
- ovarian and tumours
- aortic aneurysm leakage
- colonic tumours

Investigations should include FBC, U+Es, LFTs, blood cultures, urinalysis and AXR.

The management is similar to that of any suspected intre-abdominal sepsis – intravenous fluids, antibiotics (cefuroxime and metronidazole), anti-emetic and appropriate analgesia. patients may also have present with rectal bleeding and in this case require colonoscopy to exclude colonic carcinoma.

STATION 1.16

Assessment	Good	Adequate	Poor/not done
1 Appropriate introduction (full name and role)	☐	☐	☐
2 Candidate washes their hands using the alcohol handwash provided (no marks if candidate only expresses the need to wash if handwash is provided)	☐	☐	☐
3 Examines hands and fingernails	☐	☐	☐
4 Examines conjunctiva, tongue and fauces	☐	☐	☐
5 Examines for supraclavicular nodes	☐	☐	☐
6 Exposes abdomen and identifies laparotomy scar and stoma	☐	☐	☐
7 Palpates for liver, spleen, kidneys and other abdominal masses	☐	☐	☐
8 Percusses and auscultates abdomen	☐	☐	☐
9 Does all in a fluent, professional manner	☐	☐	☐

Clinical note for assessor

This is a 37-year-old woman who underwent a total colectomy and an ileostomy for Crohn's disease five years ago. She is currently well and in remission.

Please note – the original stoma site in the right iliac fossa has been revised. Thus the stoma is now re-formed on the left. This should not be confused with a colostomy which is normally sited in this position.

Comment

Examination of the abdomen must start with the hands for clubbing, pallor, liver palms and liver flap, followed by the conjunctiva and tongue for pallor. Supraclavicular nodes are classical sites for metastatic deposits from gastric and pancreatic cancers. Gentle abdominal palpation detects inflammation (local or generalised), organomegaly and pathological masses. Percussion detects gaseous distension and ascites, while auscultation is for bowel sounds.

Abdominal stomas may be intubated (eg gastrostomy or caecostomy) or be open (ileostomy, colostomy or ileal conduit). Cutaneous fistulae and sinuses take a number of forms but are usually the result of pathology and distinguishable from stomas by the presence of surrounding abdominal wall distortion, scarring and soilage.

STATION 1.17

Assessment	Good	Adequate	Poor/not done
1 Appropriate introduction (full name and role)	☐	☐	☐
2 Explain examination to patient and get his verbal consent	☐	☐	☐
3 Candidate washes their hands using the alcohol handwash provided (no marks if candidate only expresses the need to wash if handwash is provided)	☐	☐	☐
4 Stands patient up, pulls down his underpants and observes both inguinal regions and the scrotum	☐	☐	☐
5 Asks the patient to point out the lump, if it is tender and whether there is one on the other side	☐	☐	☐
6 Feels the lump and asks the patient to cough. Reports on the cough impulse	☐	☐	☐
7 Reduces the lump by gently squeezing the dome of the sac and using the second hand to massage the contents through the superficial inguinal ring	☐	☐	☐
8 After reduction through the ring and along the inguinal canal, places finger above the deep inguinal ring (above the midpoint of the inguinal ligament)	☐	☐	☐
9 Asks patient to cough again and reports whether it is controlled (indirect inguinal hernia) or not	☐	☐	☐
10 Examines for cough impulse on the left side	☐	☐	☐
11 Examines the testes, spermatic cord and contents of the scrotum bilaterally	☐	☐	☐

12 Tells the patient the examination is
    complete and that he can pull up .
    his underpants and thanks him   ☐   ☐   ☐

13 Is able to discuss the differential diagnosis
    of a lump in the groin   ☐   ☐   ☐

STATION 1.18

fig 1.18a – Black hairy tongue **2**, **3**, **4**, **6**
fig 1.18b – Fissured **1**, **2**, **6**
fig 1.18c – Leucoplakia **2**, **4**, **5**
fig 1.18d – Carcinoma **4**

Comment

A white patch in the mouth is called leukoplakia. Approximately 3% of white patches
undergo malignant change in five years. Biopsy is, therefore, essential. Erythroplasia
(red patches in the mouth) have a higher predilection to malignancy. Carcinoma of
the mouth is associated with smokers, and tobacco and betel nut chewers. Carcinoma
of the tongue is treated by surgery or radiotherapy; cervical nodal spread requires a
block dissection.

STATION 1.19

1 fig 1.19a: Oesophageal varices
   fig 1.19b: Raised polypoid mucosal lesion
2 (a)   (i) Oesophageal varices secondary to portal hypertension
          (ii) Gastric (antral) carcinoma
   (b) Multiple endoscopic mucosal biopsies for histological confirmation
3 (a) Cirrhosis of the liver due to alcoholic liver damage, hepatitis B or C, or Wilson's disease
   (b) Megaloblastic anaemia associated with achlorhydria
4 (a) Haematemesis, melaena
   (b) Dyspepsia, anorexia, tiredness and weight loss, melaena

Comment

Oesophageal varices are treated by endoscopic sclerotherapy, with long-term endoscopic surveillance, sclerosis of recurrences, and propranolol therapy. Nutritional and lifestyle measures are called for to halt the progression of cirrhotic change.

Gastric cancers present insidiously, with vague dyspepsia and anaemia. Dyspepsia of eight weeks' or more duration requires an endoscopic assessment. Non-ulcer dyspepsia is common, and antral mucosal biopsies invariably reveal a type II gastritis associated with *Helicobacter pylori* infection.

STATION 1.20

1 fig 1.20a: oedematous, inflamed mucosa with haemorrhage and covered with yellow exudate or slough
   fig 1.20b: sessile mucosal polyp
2 fig 1.20a: acute pseudomembranous colitis
   fig 1.20b: rectal polyp
3 (a) Long-term antibiotic therapy producing a superinfection
   (b) Rectal carcinoma
4 fig 1.20a: IV fluid and electrolyte replacement
   Stop patient's current antibiotic regime
   fig 1.20b: endoscopic excision and histological examination. If benign, place patient on colonoscopic surveillance; if malignant, surgical excision of rectum with preoperative radiotherapy

Comment

fig 1.20a: pseudomembranous colitis is a potentially lethal complication of intermittent or long-term antibiotic therapy for infective or ulcerative colitis. It is also a complication of AIDS. The causative agent is *Clostridium difficile.*

fig 1.20b: colorectal carcinoma is thought to evolve from adenomatous or dysplastic polyps and from the familial polyposis syndrome. In the latter, the entire colon is studded with polyps and, as malignant transformation is inevitable, prophylactic total colectomy is advised.

Colonoscopic biopsies would confirm the diagnosis in both cases.

STATION 1.21

1 (E) (d)
This patient has coeliac disease which causes malabsorption within the jejunum leading to folate deficiency, hypoalbuminaemia, hypocalcaemia and hypomagnesaemia. Any patient in this age group presenting with a macrocytic anaemia should be screened for coeliac disease. This should include a duodenal biopsy which will show the classical pattern of subtotal villous atrophy. Anti-endomysial antibodies are the specific immune marker in this disease.

2 (D) (e)
Patients with alcohol-related liver disease may present with a pancytopaenia, as in this case, due to the direct toxic effects of alcohol on the bone marrow. The macrocytosis may be due to the liver disease or the direct effect of the alcohol.

3 (A) (f)
All causes of upper and lower GI bleeding can present with a microcytic anaemia. However, acute bleeding is often associated with a thrombocytosis. Change in bowel habit in patients over the age of 40 requires further investigation and this patient should have a colonoscopy.

4 (F) (b)
Pernicious anaemia is associated with several autoimmune diseases particularly hypothyroidism. The macrocytosis may be due to the hypothyroidism or the B_{12} deficiency of pernicious anaemia. Severe B_{12} deficiency, as in this case, causes bone marrow suppression leading to a pancytopaenia. However, this occurs over a long period of time and leads to the grossly suppressed haemoglobin, which may often be surprisingly well tolerated. Treatment in this case should include thyroid replacement, B_{12} injections and upper GI endoscopy, as such patients are at increased risk of gastric carcinoma.

5 (C) (a)
This patient has a microcytic anaemia indicating a chronic bleeding problem but this is associated with a raised platelet count and melaena, both indicators of acute blood loss. He requires a 6 unit cross match and urgent upper GI endoscopy.

6 **(B) (c)**

Inflammatory bowel disease commonly causes a normochromic, normocytic anaemia. If associated with GI blood loss it may cause a microcytic anaemia and, rarely, terminal ileal Crohn's disease may lead to B_{12} deficiency.

STATION 1.22

1 **(E) (c)**

Carcinoma of the head of the pancreas causes an obstructive jaundice, the patient often presenting 'severely' jaundiced both clinically and biochemically.

2 **(B) (e)**

Primary biliary cirrhosis is an autoimmune disorder of the liver which principally affects middle-aged women. It has been postulated that there is a cross antigen reaction in childhood between *E. coli* and hepatocytes. Patients present with signs of chronic liver disease and may have a hepatitic jaundice.

3 **(A) (b)**

Coeliac disease is also an autoimmune disease of the small bowel. It may present at any age but principally affects young female adults. It rarely causes derangement of the liver function tests but causes general malabsorption leading to folate deficiency, hypocalcaemia, hypomagnesaemia and hypoalbuminaemia.

4 **(D) (a)**

Colonic carcinoma commonly metastasises to the liver and the skeleton. There is derangement of the liver function tests with a raised alkaline phosphatase. This may indicate both liver and bony metastases as it is produced in both tissues, but the raised calcium infers bony metastases as well.

5 **(C) (d)**

Gallstones within the lower common bile duct may produce an obstructive jaundice with an acute pancreatitis. An amylase over 1000 may be caused by an acute pancreatitis, a perforated viscus or a leaking abdominal aortic aneurysm. The low calcium is indicative of acute pancreatitis.

STATION 1.23

1 (D) (e)
Chronic viral hepatitis is the principal risk factor for developing a hepatoma. All
patients with decompensating chronic disease should be screened for a hepatoma
using the marker alpha fetoprotein and ultrasound scan. Hepatoma may be amenable
to surgical resection or radiological embolisation.

2 (C) (f)
This patient has developed liver metastases from a primary colonic carcinoma.
Although CEA is requested in many hospitals as a screening tool for colonic
carcinoma, the pick-up rate has been disappointingly low. It should be mainly used
after surgical resection as a marker of secondary disease, so that aggressive therapy
may be instituted.

3 (E) (a)
This patient has developed primary haemachromatosis, an autosomal recessive
disorder of iron metabolism. Excess iron is laid down in the liver leading to cirrhosis
and its secondary sequelae. The suntanned appearance is due to melanin excess in
the skin and not iron. Treatment is by regular venesection, some patients also
requiring the chelating agent desferrioxamine. All first degree relatives should
undergo screening.

4 (B) (c)
This patient has primary biliary cirrhosis, an autoimmune disorder of the liver which
principally affects middle-aged women. It is thought to be a cross antigen reaction
between *E.coli* and hepatocytes, as these patients have been shown to be susceptible
to *E. coli* UTIs in childhood. Immune markers of the disease include antimitochondrial
antibodies and, less commonly, anti smooth muscle and antinuclear antibodies.

5 (F) (b)
Autoimmune hepatitis (previously termed autoimmune or lupoid chronic active
hepatitits) has now been divided into two separate disorders by the different
autoantibodies present.

Type 1 is characterised by non-organ-specific autoantibodies and liver-specific
autoantibodies. Non-organ specific autoantibodies are a heterogeneous group, the
commonest being the dsDNA antibodies. The principal of these is in antismooth
muscle antibodies with anti-actin specificity. The most specific of the liver antibodies
is anti-ASGP-R (asialoglycoprotein receptor).

Type 2 is characterised by the presence of circulating antiliver/kidney microsomal
antibodies (anti-LKM), which have been subdivided into three distinct antibodies anti-
LKM 1,2 and 3.

6 **(A) (d)**

Wilson's disease is a rare autosomal recessive disorder which leads to an inability to metabolise copper normally. The copper is deposited in various sites, the liver, leading to cirrhosis, the brain, particularly the basal ganglia, and the cornea, leading to the pathgnomonic Kayser–Fleischer ring. The disorder leads to a dyskinetic syndrome or bradykinetic/rigidity syndrome (Parkinsonism). There is an associated progressive cognitive impairment. The progression of the disease may be 'retarded' by the use of oral penicillamine. All relatives should have genetic counselling and screening.

STATION 1.24

(1)	False	(7)	True
(2)	True	(8)	True
(3)	False	(9)	True
(4)	False	(10)	False
(5)	True	(11)	True
(6)	False	(12)	False

Patient (a): This patient has evidence of acute viral replication (aHBc IgM positive) and high infectivity risk (HBe Ag positive) indicating acute viral hepatitis.

Patient (b): The presence of HBs antibody shows previous exposure to the Hepatitis B virus with subsequent development of immunity. This may occur after vaccination or after the resolution of an acute infection.

Patient (c): This patient continues to express HBV DNA, which has become encoded within their own genome (HBs Ag positive). However the expression of aHBc IgG shows no ongoing viral replication. The patient remains HBe Ag positive which means they are still at high risk of passing on the infection and must be warned about sexual and drug-taking practices.

Patient (d): This patient is a chronic carrier but is at low risk of passing on the infection and does not have evidence of ongoing viral replication. However these patients are still not allowed to give blood in the UK.

STATION 1.25

1 **(E) (d)**	4 **(F) (b)**
2 **(D) (e)**	5 **(C) (a)**
3 **(A) (f)**	6 **(B) (c)**

STATION 1.26

1 fig 1.26a: Supine view of the abdomen; fig 1.26b erect antero-posterior (AP) views of the abdomen
2 Dilatation of stomach and jejunal, and ileal bowel loops (fig 1.26a), with air fluid levels (fig 1.26b)
3 Acute small bowel obstruction
4 Place patient on a 'drip and suck' regime. Assess serum urea and electrolytes and replace fluid and electrolyte deficit
   Hourly naso-gastric aspiration
   Ascertain cause of bowel obstruction and organise surgical relief if required
   Intramuscular analgesia for pain relief

Comment
Small bowel obstruction usually presents acutely, while large bowel obstruction is insidious in onset. Relief of small bowel obstruction must be immediate to prevent perforation or gangrene. Exceptions are sub-acute obstruction due to adhesions, or a bolus obstruction which may resolve with its passage. Fluid and electrolyte depletion from vomiting and third compartment loss is life-threatening and must be replaced through IV access.

STATION 1.27

1 Barium enema examination
2 Instil liquid barium into the rectum under hydrostatic pressure not exceeding 30 cm water. Tilt the patient as required to demonstrate the colon
3 A segment of colon showing an intraluminal obstruction from an intussusception of the large bowel
4 Surgical reduction of the intussusception if the bowel is viable, or resection of the involved loops of the bowel if the viability is in doubt

Comment
Intussusception is a cause of bowel obstruction in infants during weaning, but is rare in adults. It is, however, a cause of insidious bowel obstruction in AIDS and is associated with bowel lymphoma and Kaposi's sarcoma. Contrast-enhanced CT scan of the abdomen is the preferred method of diagnosing this condition in these patients who may have co-existing symptoms from the chronic enteric infections.

STATION 1.28

1 (a) **True**   (b) **False**   (c) **True**   (d) **True**   (e) **True**
This is an erect CXR showing gas below the right hemidiaphragm. The principal causes of this appearance is perforation of a hollow viscus such as bowel. Free air under the diaphragm is expected 48 hours post-laparoscopy but would indicate perforation post-ERCP. The initial management of a patient with perforation is intravenous antibiotics, eg metronidazole and cefuroxime, intravenous fluids and NG tube. This is colloquially known as 'drip and suck'. In patients unable to have operative intervention, this conservative management may allow time for the perforation to be 'walled off' and heal, if it is small and the contamination will be limited.

2 (a) **True**   (b) **False**   (c) **False**   (d) **True**   (e) **False**
This is a plain, supine film showing large bowel obstruction. Small bowel is differentiated from large bowel by the plica circulares which extend across the entire small bowel width. The large bowel is defined by the haustration of its wall. Two grossly dilated lengths of large bowel fill the length of the abdomen. Fluid levels are a feature of an erect film and are therefore not seen in this X-ray. The ground glass appearance in the right iliac fossa is produced by faecal loading. Adhesions commonly cause small bowel obstruction but are a relatively rare cause of large bowel problems. Common causes include diverticular disease, tumours, abscesses, volvulus and extrinsic compression from pelvic tumours.

3 (a) **False**   (b) **False**   (c) **True**   (d) **True**   (e) **False**
fig 1.28c is an erect CXR showing a large, probably incarcerated rolling hiatus hernia: showing stomach shadow and probable small gut loop. The 'double' left cardiac border is a result of the retrocardiac hernia. The hernia contains an air-fluid level which raises the possibility of the hernia being obstructed. Patients with a large hiatus hernia may have insidious gastrointestinal blood loss leading to a microcytic anaemia.

STATION 1.29

1 (a) **False**   (b) **True**   (c) **False**   (d) **True**   (e) **True**
This is a barium swallow showing a long, smooth stricture, consistent with a benign lesion. Common causes are oesophageal reflux and corrosives. Presbyoesophagus, ('cork screw oesophagus') is a benign condition of old age and is a diagnosis made on video-fluoroscopy; it must be differentiated from malignancy.

2 (a) **True**   (b) **False**   (c) **False**   (d) **False**   (e) **True**
This barium swallow shows a grossly dilated lower oesophagus with a classical 'bird beak' deformity in the distal segment. There is 'abundant' food residue within this dilated segment. These appearances are consistent with achalasia. This is an idiopathic disorder, which is caused by an aganglionic segment of the lower oesophagus, (similar to Hirschsprung's disease of the rectum). It is an important diagnosis as it is a premalignant condition.

3 (a) **False**   (b) **False**   (c) **True**   (d) **False**   (e) **True**
On comparing the stricture in the barium swallow in (1) and this examination, the strictured segment is very irregular and is diagnostic of a carcinoma. Oesophageal carcinoma is related to cigarette smoking, heavy alcohol intake and spicy foods. Predisposing conditions include achalasia, tylosis, Plummer–Vinson syndrome and Barret's oesophagus.

STATION 1.30

1 (a) **True**   (b) **True**   (c) **False**   (d) **True**   (e) **False**

This is a barium meal and follow through (into the small bowel) study showing a large 3 cm ulcer crater on the posterior wall of the body of the stomach (fig 1.30ai). The smooth margins indicate its probable benign nature. There is almost complete loss of the normal gastric rugae (folds) which indicates gastric atrophy and raises the possibility of pernicious anaemia. In the follow through there is evidence of incidental duodenal and jejunal diverticulae and some gallstones are also outlined.

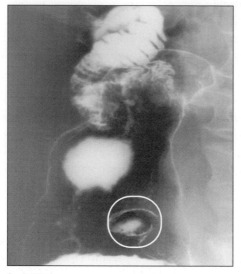

fig 1.30ai

2 (a) **False**   (b) **False**   (c) **True**   (d) **False**   (e) **True**

This is a barium meal showing a large ulcer on the lesser curvature of the antrum and body of the stomach. Its irregular margins (comparing it to the previous example) indicate it is probably a malignant ulcer. Carcinoma of the stomach is associated with the presence of *H. pylori* and pernicious anaemia. It is therefore advisable that early eradication therapy is given to younger patients presenting with peptic ulcer disease and that patients with pernicious anaemia have endoscopic follow up.

3 (a) **True**   (b) **False**   (c) **True**   (d) **True**   (e) **True**

This is a barium meal and follow through showing a grossly shrunken, poorly distended stomach. The oesophagus and duodenum are within normal limits. This appearance is due to diffuse mucosal infiltration by a gastric carcinoma. This appearance is termed a 'leather bottle' stomach or linitis plastica.

STATION 1.31

1 (a) **True**   (b) **False**   (c) **True**   (d) **False**   (e) **False**
This is a barium enema taken with the patient lying on their right as witnessed by
the fluid levels. The study shows multiple diverticulae throughout the colon.
Diverticular disease is related to a poor fibre, western diet and is rarely seen in black
Africans. The disorder is unrelated to inflammatory bowel disease.

2 (a) **False**   (b) **True**   (c) **False**   (d) **False**   (e) **True**
This is a double contrast barium study showing loss of the haustral pattern in the
distal two-thirds of the transverse colon and the descending colon. This appearance is
termed 'lead piping' and is a feature of ulcerative colitis. The small indentations are
pseudopolyps and not diverticulae. The incidence of inflammatory bowel disease is
similar in the two sexes. The incidence of colonic carcinoma is greatly increased in
patients with ulcerative colitis for 10 years or more and they should be under
colonoscopic surveillance.

3 (a) **True**   (b) **False**   (c) **True**   (d) **False**   (e) **True**
This is a double contrast study showing a classical 'apple core' stricture of the
transverse colon (fig 1.31C). This appearance is classical of colonic cancer. Patients
present with weight loss, change in bowel habit and bleeding and mucus per rectum.
Colonic carcomoma usually presents in the 6th to 7th decade.

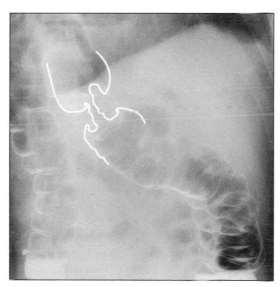

fig 1.31c

STATION 1.32

(A) Liver

(F) Right crus of the diaphragm

(B) Spleen

(G) Liver metastases

(C) Lumbar vertebra

(D) Abdominal aorta

(E) Ribs

STATION 1.33

1 (a)This is an ERCP (endoscopic retrograde cholangiopancreatogram).

(b) It shows a markedly dilated common bile duct and biliary tree and a filling defect at the lower end of the bile duct. No gallstones are identified. At operation, a carcinoma of the ampulla of Vater was identified and resected.

2 (a) This is a selective coeliac axis arteriogram which is principally used to delineate small tumours of the pancreas, eg insulinomas.

(b) The arteriogram shows normal splenic, left gastric and hepatic arteries but the gastroduodenal and pancreaticoduodenal arteries show a blush at their distal ends, with encasement and narrowing of the pancreaticoduodenal artery proximally. These appearances suggest a pancreatic carcinoma.

3 (a) This is an ultrasound scan of the liver.

(b) Ultrasound is a relatively simple, safe, non-invasive procedure which is extremely useful in visualising the intra-abdominal viscera. Indications for its use include hepatobiliary disease, particularly the investigation of jaundice. Structures that may be visualised include liver metastases, gallstones and other causes of obstruction of the hepatobiliary tree. Pancreatic views are technically a little more difficult and ultrasound has been superceded in many respects by CT scanning to visualise the pancreas. Other intra-abdominal indications include investigations of any mass, visualising the renal tract and the pelvic organs. Ultrasound may be used to define an aortic aneurysm but in the acute situation dissection can only be truly excluded at operation or by CT scan of the abdomen. This scan shows multiple, heterogeneous lesions within the liver, consistent with metastases.

4 (a) This is a right decubitus view of a barium enema showing the classical appearances of the twisted neck of a sigmoid volvulus.

(b)The sigmoid colon has become twisted with resulting gross dilatation. The initial treatment is to attempt to pass a flatus tube across the twisted segment into the obstructed sigmoid loop. If this is successful, the flatus tube should be left in for 24 to 48 hours. If this fails, a limited barium enema should be attempted which may cause the volvulus to untwist. If both of these manoeuvres are unsuccessful, urgent surgical intervention is required, usually involving sigmoid colectomy.

5 (a) This is an erect CXR showing a calcified mass in the right upper quadrant.
(b) This patient had a hydatid cyst, but many chronic conditions produce calcification within the liver, eg tuberculosis; arterio-venous anomalies; aneurysms, hepatoma and metastases.

STATION 1.34

This woman has a duodenal ulcer which is proven to be associated with *Helicobacter pylori.* She should therefore be started on a course of eradication and ulcer-healing therapy. As yet there is no single agreed regimen. Eradication therapy combines one or two antibiotics with an antisecretory drug. For full ulcer healing the antisecretory drug may need to be continued for a further 1–2 months. The regimen chosen must be relatively 'user friendly' as often the biggest problem is poor patient adherence. Recently therefore, one-week regimes have been advocated using higher doses of the drugs.

Suggested combinations are shown below. (as in *Prescriber's Journal* 1996, Vol.36 No. 3.)

One week:
Triple therapy – eradication rates vary from 80–90%.
Amoxycillin 750 mg tds + metronidazole 400 mg tds + ranitidine 300 mg nocte
Amoxycillin 500 mg tds + metronidazole 400 mg tds + omeprazole 20 mg bd or
ILansoprazole 30 mg bd
Amoxycillin 1 g bd + clarithromycin 500 mg bd + omeprazole 20 mg bd or
lansoprazole 30 mg bd
Clarithromycin 250 mg bd + metronidazole 400 mg bd + omeprazole 20 mg bd or
Lansoprazole 30 mg bd

Two weeks:
Dual therapy – eradication rates vary from 60–80%
Amoxycillin 1 g bd + omeprazole 20mg bd or lansoprazole 30 mg bd
Clarithromycin 500 mg tds + omeprazole 40 mg mane

The correct prescription should be filled in with any of the regimens suggested above, ensuring the patient details are all correct, the drugs, doses and frequencies are clearly stated and the duration of therapy is written below. The prescription must be signed, with your name printed and dated.

STATION 1.35

1 **False**

He is likely to be in a catabolic state due to sepsis and multiple trauma.

2 **False**

He has a disproportionately raised creatinine compared to his urea. This suggests he has renal cellular damage, as well as any prerenal impairment.

3 **True**

To calculate his corrected calcium: calcium + (standard albumin [40 mmol/l] – serum albumin) x 0.02 = 1.9 + ([40–19] x 0.02) = 2.12 mmol/l)

4 **False**

40 mmol is the normal daily requirement. This patient has marked hypokalaemia and therefore requires 100–200 mmol.

5 **True**

If peripheral or central venous access is becoming difficult, the insulin maybe given in the TPN bag. However, under normal circumstances, an IV sliding scale insulin regime should be maintained.

6 **True**

Although he has a low albumin he cannot have a high protein concentration in his TPN because of his renal impairment.

7 **False**

His BMI: weight (kg)/height (m^2) 2–80/3.24 = 24.69 (normal = 20–28)

8 **True**

He can receive all his fluid replacements through the TPN.

9 **False**

He will require increased calories because of the catabolic effects of the sepsis.

10 **True**

Although a 'dedicated' line is better.

STATION 1.36

1 **False**   2 **True**   3 **False**

Instrument A is a sigmoidoscope used to view the first 10–25 cm of distal large bowel. It is used to view the bowel mucosa to exclude local inflammation, tumours and bleeding sites. Biopsy forceps may be inserted through the sigmoidoscope in order to biopsy mucosa or tumours. Sigmoidoscopy should be nothing more than 'uncomfortable' and it is very rare to even give sedation.

4 **False**   5 **True**   6 **True**

Instrument B is a Sengstaken–Blakemore tube. Although endoscopy has allowed direct access to sources of both upper and lower gastrointestinal bleeding, the Sengstaken tube may still play a vital role in containment of a bleeding site in the lower oesophagus or stomach. It is particularly useful in bleeding from oesophageal varices. A tennis ball or similar soft object is often attached to the proximal end of the tube, cushioned and tied against the face, to stop the patient swallowing the entire tube! After an initial examination, sigmoidoscopy precedes proctoscopy to avoid misinterpretation of any hyperaemia produced in the rectum by the proctoscope: local perianal conditions can also be undertaken through the proctoscope, with the knowledge that proximal rectal pathology has already been excluded. Proctoscopy must be undertaken routinely after any sigmoidoscopy.

7 **True**   8 **False**   9 **False**

Instrument C is a proctoscope used to look at local disease within the rectum. It may be used with a sigmoidoscope but it is often used independently. Sigmoidoscopy usually precedes protoscopy so that erythema produced by the latter is not misinterpreted as inflammation, and that therapeutic measures, such as the injection of piles, can be undertaken, knowing that there are no contraindictions pertaining to the rectum.

10 **False**   11 **True**   12 **False**

Instrument D is a liver biopsy needle. The patient must be able to lie flat on their back and hold their breath for approximately 10 seconds to allow the biopsy to be taken. Apart from being unable to do either of these, other contraindications include local skin sepsis, deranged clotting or thrombocytopaenia, gross ascites and extrahepatic cholestasis. The patient should have a FBC and clotting screen prior to the procedure and full informed consent should be obtained. The procedure is usually performed with local anaesthetic.

13 **False**   14 **True**   15 **False**

Instrument E is an endoscope used to view the upper and lower bowel. It has now been shown that coeliac disease may be diagnosed from duodenal biopsies and has made the use of the Crosby–Kugler capsule unnecessary. ERCP is performed through a slightly modified endoscope. Pneumomediastinum is a relatively rare complication of an upper GI endoscopy. It may arise due to force being applied to the endoscope or through biopsying areas of the oesophagus, causing tears in the mucosa. Small tears will cause few problems and heal over with no further intervention. Large tears however need surgical repair.

16 **True**   17 **True**   18 **False**

Instrument F is a nasogastric tube used to feed and hydrate patients who are having difficulty maintaining their nutritional input. This may be due to a decreased level of consciousness or mechanical swallowing problems, both of which may occur in a stroke patient. The feeding of patients using the gut is known as enteral feeding. Parenteral feeding is the use of specialised feeding lines inserted into a vein. The tube is radio-opaque to allow its position to be seen on a chest radiograph. Its position may be checked clinically by pushing 50 ml of air from a syringe down the tube while listening with a stethoscope over the stomach, or by aspirating fluid back along the tube and then testing with litmus paper to see if it is acidic.

Chapter 2:
Neurology and Psychiatry
Answers

Chapter 2

Neurology and Psychiatry Answers

STATION 2.1

Patient history

I am 21 years old and have been well until about four months ago, when I started the oral contraceptive pill. Since then I have had a number of severe, generalised headaches. They seem to come on at any time, but especially when I have red wine. They are 'thumping' and I often get a strange feeling about 2 or 3 hours before they really start. The feeling is like muzziness and tiredness.

The headaches last about 24 hours before they finally go. I have to take four aspirin to get any relief. The headaches are made worse by loud noise but I haven't noticed that they are any worse in the morning or when crying, laughing or straining. They do ease a little if I lie down in a quiet room. I get flashing lights in my eyes, and any bright light hurts my eyes. I don't get a stiff neck. I am often very sick with the headaches and vomit throughout the period of worst pain. I have never had headaches before; no-one in my family has migraine.

Apart from this problem I am well and haven't had any blackouts, fits, weakness or loss of feeling in my limbs. My speech is not affected. I am very worried about the possibility of a brain tumour. Also I am having to take time off work which is a problem.

Assessment	Good	Adequate	Poor/not done
1 Appropriate introduction (full name and role)	☐	☐	☐
2 Explains purpose of interview	☐	☐	☐
3 Establishes onset of symptoms	☐	☐	☐
4 Establishes the characteristics of the headache:			
Site		☐	☐
Radiation		☐	☐
Nature/severity		☐	☐
Relieving factors		☐	☐
Exacerbating factors		☐	☐
Precipitating factors		☐	☐
5 Establishes associated symptoms:			
Meningism		☐	☐
Nausea and vomiting		☐	☐
Warning aura		☐	☐
Visual disturbances		☐	☐
6 Excludes previous family history of migraine	☐	☐	☐
7 Elicits patient's concerns and responds sensitively	☐	☐	☐
8 Uses an appropriate questioning technique	☐	☐	☐
9 Avoids or explains jargon	☐	☐	☐
10 Summarises history back to the patient, including concerns	☐	☐	☐
11 Systematic, organised approach	☐	☐	☐

Diagnosis

Migraine attacks.

Comment

Treatment of migraine: once precipitants have been identified and excluded, treatment may be divided into symptom relief and prophylaxis.

Symptom relief: appropriate analgesics should be used to relieve the headache. Patients should be advised to start with simple analgesia such as aspirin and paracetamol and then move up the analgesic ladder to opiates such as codeine phosphate. Oral analgesia may be hampered by vomiting and it may be necessary to give the analgesia by intramuscular or per rectal routes. Anti-emetics such as metoclopramide and domperidone are commonly used. 5-HT agonists such as ergotamine and sumatriptan may be used in acute attacks and relieve the pain and nausea in about two-thirds of patients.

Prophylaxis: this should be offered to patients having more than two attacks per month. Treatments include beta blockers, 5-HT antagonists (5-HT agonists are used in acute episodes), cyproheptadine, pizotifen, methysergide and calcium antagonists.

The many drugs used in treatment is an indication of the uncertainty of the causes of migraine. The drugs act on various receptors, including those for 5-HT, calcium channels and histamine. Their various actions include vasoconstriction, membrane stabilisation and reducing sympathetic outflow.

Answers

STATION 2.2

Patient history

I am 19 years old and am studying for my final school examinations. I was well until about three months ago, when I started to get increasingly severe headaches. They are mainly on the right side of my forehead, radiating to the back of the head. At first it was a dull ache, but now the headaches are extremely painful, and aspirin or paracetamol don't help. The headaches are almost constant but are much worse in the early morning when I wake up and when I am straining on the toilet, coughing or laughing.

In the last few weeks I have felt dreadful – very tired and out of sorts, with no energy. I have been nauseated and have been vomiting with blurring of my vision. In fact, I can't go on revising for my examinations. In the last two days I have had two blackouts, and have woken up feeling very battered and bruised. I have also wet myself. Over the last week my left hand and arm have felt weak, and I have dropped a few things.

I am really worried about what might be wrong and whether I can carry on with my studies.

Assessor: Please ask the student – 'What course of action would you now take?' (patient requires urgent admission).

Assessment	Good	Adequate	Poor/not done
1 Appropriate introduction (full name and role)	☐	☐	☐
2 Explains purpose of interview	☐	☐	☐
3 Establishes the duration of symptoms	☐	☐	☐
4 Establishes the characteristics of the headache:			
Site		☐	☐
Nature/severity		☐	☐
Radiation		☐	☐
Relieving factors		☐	☐
Exacerbating factors		☐	☐
Precipitating factors		☐	☐

5 Establishes the associated symptoms:

   Nausea and vomiting ☐ ☐

   Blurring of vision ☐ ☐

6 Establishes history of associated neurological
   symptoms: ☐ ☐

   Episode of blackout ☐ ☐

   Mild weakness in left arm ☐ ☐

7 Establishes systemic symptoms:

   Lethargy ☐ ☐

   Malaise ☐ ☐

   Weight loss ☐ ☐

8 Elicits patient's concerns and responds
   sensitively ☐ ☐ ☐

9 Uses an appropriate questioning
   technique ☐ ☐ ☐

10 Summarises history back to the patient ☐ ☐ ☐

11 Systematic organised approach ☐ ☐ ☐

12 Makes a reasonable attempt at the
   diagnosis ☐ ☐ ☐

13 When asked states that the patient needs
   urgent admission ☐ ☐ ☐

Answers

Diagnosis

Space-occupying lesion leading to raised intracranial pressure and localising signs, ie left arm weakness and seizures.

STATION 2.3

Patient history

I am 23 years old and have always kept well but while I was at work today I developed the worst headache in the world. I feel very frightened and upset about it. I work as a hairdresser and while I was cutting someone's hair about three hours ago, this terrible headache suddenly came on out of the blue. It was like a clap of thunder going off in my head. The pain is mainly at the back of my head but doesn't seem to radiate anywhere else. I have felt dizzy and unwell since the headache came on and I've vomited two or three times. Nothing seems to be making the headache any better, and I don't think it could possibly get any worse! My neck feels stiff, and I can't look into the light because it hurts my eyes. I haven't had any cold, sore throat or cough.

I've never had headaches before but I remember my mother telling me that my grandmother had kidney problems and died in childbirth, aged 34, of a bleed in the brain. Might something like this be happening to me?

Assessment	Good	Adequate	Poor/not done
1 Appropriate introduction (full name and role)	☐	☐	☐
2 Explains purpose of interview	☐	☐	☐
3 Establishes the duration and onset of symptoms	☐	☐	☐
4 Is sensitive to the fact patient is in severe distress; mentions the need for analgesia and antiemetic	☐	☐	☐
5 Establishes the characteristics of the headache:			
Site		☐	☐
Nature/severity		☐	☐
Relieving factors		☐	☐
Exacerbating factors		☐	☐
Precipitating factors		☐	☐

6 Establishes associated symptoms:

   Neck stiffness   ☐   ☐

   Nausea and vomiting   ☐   ☐

   Mild photophobia   ☐   ☐

7 Excludes fever and symptoms of upper
   and lower respiratory tract infection   ☐   ☐   ☐

8 Establishes family history of
   cerebrovascular and renal disease   ☐   ☐   ☐

9 Excludes previous history of headaches
   specifically migraine   ☐   ☐   ☐

10 Uses an appropriate questioning
   technique   ☐   ☐   ☐

11 Avoids or explains jargon   ☐   ☐   ☐

12 Summarises history back to the patient   ☐   ☐   ☐

13 Systematic organised approach   ☐   ☐   ☐

14 Makes a reasonable attempt at the
   diagnosis   ☐   ☐   ☐

SP to mark

15 The student showed empathy   ☐   ☐   ☐

Answers

Diagnosis
Subarachnoid haemorrhage probably secondary to the rupture of a Berry aneurysm.

STATION 2.4

Patient history

I am 17 years old and still at school. I have always been well but I have had four or five funny turns in the last couple of months. At least two of these were only 48 hours apart. The turns can come on at any time but I think I know when they are about to happen because I get strange feelings in my hands and feet, as if they were on fire. I get dreamy-like visions in front of my eyes. I don't remember anything about the turns but I know I become unconscious. My mother saw it happen the last time and said I fell to the floor, and began shaking, and grunting very loudly. I was frothing at the mouth and wet myself, too. The turn lasted three or four minutes and then got better. When I woke up I felt battered and bruised, and very sleepy. My mother put me to bed, and I slept for three hours. When I woke up I felt much better but had a bit of a headache.

I've never had any epileptic fits before, although my mother says I had three or four fever fits when I was a baby. As far as I know, no-one in my family has epilepsy. Apart from this I am very well and haven't had any other symptoms in the last few months. I have never had a head injury, and I am not taking any medicines. I drink less than five units of alcohol in a month. I don't smoke or use recreational drugs.

I am very frightened about what is happening to me and how my life will be affected. Will I still be able to go to University?

Assessment	Good	Adequate	Poor/not done
1 Appropriate introduction (full name and role)	☐	☐	☐
2 Explains the purpose of the interview	☐	☐	☐
3 Establishes the duration and frequency of the symptoms	☐	☐	☐

4 Establishes the characteristics of
   the 'funny turns':

   Aura – warning symptoms ☐ ☐

   Memory of turns ☐ ☐

   Witness accounts; limb shaking ☐ ☐

   Post-ictal symptoms and duration ☐ ☐

   Aassociated tongue biting ☐ ☐

   Incontinence of urine ☐ ☐

   Facial plethora ☐ ☐

   Loss of consciousness ☐ ☐

5 Excludes other neurological symptoms:

   Headaches ☐ ☐

   Permanent motor and sensory deficit ☐ ☐

   Speech ☐ ☐

   Visual and hearing loss ☐ ☐

   Dizziness ☐ ☐

6 Excludes other systemic symptoms ☐ ☐ ☐

7 Establishes alcohol, cigarette and illicit
   drug history ☐ ☐ ☐

8 Excludes previous/family history of
   epilepsy, eg febrile convulsions as a child ☐ ☐ ☐

9 Excludes previous history of head injury ☐ ☐ ☐

10 Elicits patient's concerns and responds
    sensitively ☐ ☐ ☐

11 Uses an appropriate questioning technique ☐ ☐ ☐

12 Avoids or explains jargon ☐ ☐ ☐

13 Summarises history back to the patient,
    including concerns ☐ ☐ ☐

14 Systematic and organised approach ☐ ☐ ☐

15 Makes a reasonable attempt at the
    diagnosis ☐ ☐ ☐

Answers

Diagnosis

Recent onset of idiopathic epilepsy.

Comment

Management of epilepsy: patients presenting with seizures need to have a full metabolic screen, CT head scan and EEG to exclude other causes of seizures prior to a diagnosis of idiopathic epilepsy being made. Routine blood tests should include FBC, U+Es, corrected calcium and magnesium. CT head scan and EEG will exclude other underlying causes such as space-occupying lesions. Once the diagnosis of idiopathic epilepsy has been made the patient should be advised against driving a motor vehicle and taking part in certain occupations, such as operating machinery. A patient may drive a car if fit free for one year or more, or, if they have only suffered nocturnal seizures for three years. Many of the anticonvulsants used in the treatment of epilepsy have unpleasant side-effects. Patients should be told about the side-effects and then, depending on the frequency of seizures and the effects on the patient's lifestyle, treatment should be commenced.

STATION 2.5

Patient history

I am 24 years old and I have always kept fit and well. About four months ago I began to get increasing weakness of my legs and arms, particularly the arms. It gets worse the more I repeat something, such as chopping or cutting food. I have noticed that my speech is becoming strange, too, as if I had a cold. It is also increasingly difficult to swallow and chew things the longer a meal goes on. The main problem that made me go to the doctor was double vision, which is getting so bad that I can't read the paper, watch television or drive a car. My husband has said that my eyes look droopy.

I don't have any other symptoms. My muscle tone has not changed and I have had no shaking, wasting away or twitching. I can feel things quite normally. I am very concerned about what is happening. Have I had a stroke? Have I got something incurable?

Assessment	Good	Adequate	Poor/not done
1 Appropriate introduction (full name and role)	☐	☐	☐
2 Explains the purpose of the interview	☐	☐	☐
3 Establishes the duration of the symptoms	☐	☐	☐
4 Establishes the pattern of weakness, ie global weakness affecting all four limbs (upper more than lower)	☐	☐	☐
5 Characterises the weakness: increases with fatigue	☐	☐	☐
6 Excludes:			
Wasting		☐	☐
Fasciculation		☐	☐
Change in tone of the limbs		☐	☐
7 Establishes associated problems with:			
Swallowing		☐	☐
Eating		☐	☐
Speech		☐	☐

8 Establishes history of visual problems ☐ ☐ ☐

9 Excludes sensory symptoms, parasthesiae
   and numbness ☐ ☐ ☐

10 Excludes other neurological symptoms:

   Fits ☐ ☐

   Loss of consciousness ☐ ☐

   Headaches ☐ ☐

   Tremor ☐ ☐

11 Excludes other systemic symptoms ☐ ☐ ☐

12 Elicits patient's concerns and responds
   sensitively ☐ ☐ ☐

13 Uses an appropriate questioning technique ☐ ☐ ☐

14 Avoids or explains jargon ☐ ☐ ☐

15 Summarises history back to the patient
   including concerns ☐ ☐ ☐

16 Systematic and organised approach ☐ ☐ ☐

17 Makes a reasonable attempt at the
   diagnosis ☐ ☐ ☐

Patient to mark

18 The doctor was empathic ☐ ☐ ☐

Diagnosis

Myasthenia gravis.

Comment

Myasthenia gravis: this scenario can be difficult for the undergraduate but shows the importance of taking a good history.

Myasthenia is a relatively uncommon autoimmune disorder that affects women slightly more than men. It is due to an autoantibody directed against the postsynaptic part of the acetylcholine receptor and is characterised by fatiguable muscle weakness, that is weakness which worsens with repetition of an action (eg chewing of food).

The principal treatments in this disorder are the anticholinesterases, pyridostigmine and neostigmine. In more severe cases, immunosuppression, with prednisolone and azathioprine, is also used. Cyclophosphamide, methotrexate and cyclosporin are used in resistant cases, and where steroids and azathioprine are poorly tolerated.

In young patients with autoantibodies, thymectomy is advocated as up to 60% of these patients have an abnormal thymus gland, including thymoma. Thymectomy in older patients, or those without autoantibodies, has not been shown significantly to change the natural course of their disease.

STATION 2.6

Patient history

I am a 62-year-old retired lorry driver. I am being treated for blood pressure and gout. I was well until about six months ago, since when I have lost 15 kg and have become increasingly weak. I am right-handed, and my left hand has become shrivelled, as if all the muscles had been sucked out. The right hand is getting weaker and I can't hold a knife or fork in it. My legs are weak but I can still walk about 10 to 20 m. The weakness seems to spread up the affected limbs. Sometimes I have noticed that the muscles in my arms seem to twitch on their own.

My speech has changed recently and I am finding it increasingly difficult to eat. The food comes back up, often out of my nose, which I find very upsetting. I choke on both solids and liquids and this is not helping my weight loss. I am feeling very frightened about what might be wrong. I am upset that this has happened so soon after I retired.

I have not had any visual problems or any headaches, loss of consciousness, fits or other neurological symptoms. My bowels and micturition have been normal and I am relatively well otherwise.

I smoked 20 cigarettes per day until 10 years ago and I drink 20 units of alcohol per week, mainly whisky.

Assessment	Good	Adequate	Poor/not done
1 Appropriate introduction (full name and role)	☐	☐	☐
2 Explains the purpose of the interview	☐	☐	☐
3 Establishes the duration and progression of the illness	☐	☐	☐
4 Establishes the character of the weakness	☐	☐	☐
5 Establishes wasting associated with fasciculation	☐	☐	☐
6 Establishes the nature of the swallowing problems and associated speech problems	☐	☐	☐

7 Excludes visual, hearing and
comprehension problems ☐ ☐ ☐

8 Excludes other general neurological
symptoms:

Headache ☐ ☐

Fits ☐ ☐

Loss of consciousness ☐ ☐

9 Excludes other systemic illness, in
particular ensures normal sphincter
control and malignant symptoms:

Methargy ☐ ☐

Malaise ☐ ☐

Loss of appetite ☐ ☐

10 Establishes smoking, alcohol and
occupation history ☐ ☐ ☐

11 Elicits patient's concerns and responds
sensitively ☐ ☐ ☐

12 Uses an appropriate questioning
technique ☐ ☐ ☐

13 Avoids or explains jargon ☐ ☐ ☐

14 Summarises history back to patient,
including concerns ☐ ☐ ☐

15 Systematic organised approach ☐ ☐ ☐

16 Makes a reasonable attempt at the
diagnosis ☐ ☐ ☐

Patient to mark

17 It was easy to talk to this student ☐ ☐ ☐

Diagnosis
Motor neurone disease, with both bulbar and corticospinal symptoms.

STATION 2.7

Patient history

I am 24 years old and a professional footballer. I have always been fit and well until about two months ago, when I started getting visual problems and funny feelings in my hands and feet. I had a weird episode six months ago, when I was playing in a match. Suddenly the whole world went hazy and I had to come off the field. The problem had gone by the next day, so I didn't pay much attention to it. Then six to eight weeks ago when I was training, the ball felt spongy on the end of my boot, and I found it difficult to grip my knife and fork. Things have been getting worse ever since. I can't drive the car because I can't feel the pedals or the steering wheel. I haven't been able to use the train because my feet feel so strange – like cotton wool with pins and needles. My vision has been blurred on and off during the last month, and I've had a dull pain behind my eyes.

In spite of these strange sensations, I have not had any weakness in my arms and legs and there has been no wasting, twitching or shaking. I haven't had any other neurological symptoms. I don't smoke. I drink five to ten units of alcohol a week and don't take any medicines. Apart from these problems I am well, and have never had any serious illnesses.

I am very worried about what might be wrong. I can't play football in this state and am scared that I am going to have to give it up.

Assessment	Good	Adequate	Poor/not done
1 Appropriate introduction (full name and role)	☐	☐	☐
2 Explains the purpose of the interview	☐	☐	☐
3 Establishes the duration of the symptoms	☐	☐	☐
4 Establishes distal/glove and stocking distribution of sensory symptoms	☐	☐	☐
5 Excludes associated motor problems:			
Wasting		☐	☐
Fasciculation		☐	☐
Tremor		☐	☐
6 Establishes retro-orbital pain and visual loss	☐	☐	☐

7 Excludes general neurological symptoms:

Loss of consciousness ☐ ☐

Headaches ☐ ☐

Fits ☐ ☐

Dizziness ☐ ☐

8 Excludes loss of higher functions:

Swallowing ☐ ☐

Speech ☐ ☐

Comprehension ☐ ☐

Hearing loss ☐ ☐

9 Excludes other risk factors for sensory neuropathy:

Diabetes ☐ ☐

Alcohol ☐ ☐

Medications ☐ ☐

10 Excludes other systemic illness:

Weight loss ☐ ☐

Malaise ☐ ☐

GI and GU symptoms ☐ ☐

11 Elicits patient's concerns and responds with sensitivity ☐ ☐ ☐

12 Uses an appropriate questioning technique ☐ ☐ ☐

13 Avoids or explains jargon ☐ ☐ ☐

14 Summarises history back to the patient, including concerns ☐ ☐ ☐

15 Systematic, organised approach ☐ ☐ ☐

16 Is able to name the three investigations correctly ☐ ☐ ☐

17 Does all in a fluent, professional manner ☐ ☐ ☐

Patient to mark

18 The doctor was empathic   ☐   ☐   ☐

Diagnosis

Peripheral sensory neuropathy and visual disturbance secondary to demyelinating disease (principally multiple sclerosis).

Investigations

1 Lumbar puncture to confirm the presence of oligoclonal bands in the CSF
2 MRI of the brain stem and cervical cord – to establish the presence of areas of demyelination: plaques
3 Visual evoked responses
4 Clinical examination should include:
   • Fundoscopy to exclude other causes of visual problems and establish the presence of optic atrophy
   • BM stix and urinalysis

STATION 2.8

Patient history

I am 54 years old and work as an electrician. I have diabetes and high blood pressure. I don't use insulin for my diabetes. Yesterday, while I was out shopping, my left arm and leg went limp and dead, and the left side of my face felt droopy. I had no warning of this, and no headache or blackout. I fell to the floor and had to be helped up. I could understand what people were saying to me but I couldn't talk, even though I knew what I wanted to say. The problems went away after 30 or 40 minutes, and I didn't let the ambulance men take me to hospital because I thought it was a waste of everyone's time. I haven't had any problems overnight, and I feel back to normal today.

I have had high blood pressure for ten years and I've been diabetic for the last five. I've never had a mini stroke or any other stroke, and I've never had any problems with my heart or the circulation in my legs and feet. I had my cholesterol done in the diabetic clinic on my first visit, and they said it was slightly above normal but nothing to worry too much about. My father and brother both died in their 50s of heart and stroke problems. I am anxious that this is going to happen to me.

I've put on a lot of weight since I got divorced three years ago, and I now weigh about 92 kg. My height is 1.72 m. I eat all the wrong foods, and I drink five or six pints of beer a night. I still smoke 30 cigarettes a day. I have missed my last two diabetic clinic appointments and never test my blood or urine. I don't take any exercise, although I was a keen swimmer when young. I am concerned that I don't have enough will-power to change my lifestyle.

Assessment	Good	Adequate	Poor/not done
1 Appropriate introduction (full name and role)	☐	☐	☐
2 Explains purpose of interview	☐	☐	☐
3 Establishes the nature of the 'strange turn':			
Global weakness of left upper and lower limbs		☐	☐
Left-sided facial palsy		☐	☐
Expressive dysphasia/no Receptive problems.		☐	☐

Complete resolution with no recurrence since ☐ ☐

5 Excludes headache, loss of consciousness, fits ☐ ☐

6 Excludes history of similar episodes ☐ ☐

7 Establishes the risk factors for transient ischaemic episode:

Family history of atherosclerotic disease ☐ ☐

Previous history of stroke, IHD, PVD ☐ ☐

Hyperlipidaemia ☐ ☐

Smoking ☐ ☐

Hypertension ☐ ☐

Alcohol excess ☐ ☐

Cardiac arrhythmia and valvular disease ☐ ☐

General lifestyle ☐ ☐

Exercise ☐ ☐

Diet ☐ ☐

Weight ☐ ☐

8 Explains the diagnosis in a clear, jargon-free manner ☐ ☐ ☐

9 Explains to the patient lifestyle changes that need to be considered ☐ ☐ ☐

10 Elicits patient's concerns and responds sensitively ☐ ☐ ☐

11 Uses an appropriate questioning technique ☐ ☐ ☐

12 Avoids asking leading questions ☐ ☐ ☐

13 Checks understanding of proposed changes ☐ ☐ ☐

14 Systematic, organised approach ☐ ☐ ☐

15 Invites patient questions and answers appropriately ☐ ☐ ☐

SP to mark

16 The student was empathic and non-judgemental	☐	☐	☐

Diagnosis

Transient ischaemic attack (TIA) causing a left hemiparesis, expressive aphasia and a left facial palsy.

Comment

This patient has a very strong family history of premature atherosclerotic-related death. He has several primary risk factors for stroke including hypertension, diabetes (which is probably poorly controlled), cigarette smoking and excess alcohol intake. He has a high BMI of 31.1 and a sedentary lifestyle. He has now suffered a TIA.

The following management should be instituted.

- Encouragement to stop smoking, lose weight and start gentle exercise programme
- Review by dietician – diabetic, low fat, weight-losing diet
- Ensure blood pressure control
- Review by hospital diabetologist
- Addition of aspirin and dipyridamole SR as secondary prophylaxis
- Review in hospital outpatient department for:
  Duplex USS carotids
  CXR and ECG
  Echocardiogram
  Possible counselling about divorce and depression

Answers

STATION 2.9

Assessment	Good	Adequate	Poor/not done
1 Appropriate introduction (full name and role)	☐	☐	☐
2 Explains purpose of examination and gains verbal consent	☐	☐	☐
3 Candidate washes their hands using the alcohol handwash provided (no marks if candidate only expresses the need to wash if handwash is provided)	☐	☐	☐
4 Observes patient from the end of the bed commenting on the presence/absence of:			
Wasting of limbs		☐	☐
Fasciculation		☐	☐
Signs of stroke and other neurological disease		☐	☐
Cranial nerve lesions		☐	☐
5 Returns to the bedside and reassesses 'bulk' of the upper limbs – commenting on presence/absence of wasting/ fasciculation	☐	☐	☐
6 Makes an appropriate assessment of tone in the upper limbs	☐	☐	☐
7 Assesses power of:			
Shoulder abduction		☐	☐
Shoulder adduction		☐	☐
Elbow flexion		☐	☐
Wrist dorsiflexion		☐	☐
Wrist palmar flexion		☐	☐
Finger abduction		☐	☐
Thumb opposition		☐	☐
Thumb abduction		☐	☐

8 In all muscle groups, uses appropriate
   technique and always compares one side
   with the other   ☐   ☐   ☐

9 Attempts to assess co-ordination   ☐   ☐   ☐

10 Assesses the upper limb reflexes – using
   appropriate technique and comparing
   left and right   ☐   ☐   ☐

11 Assesses:

   Biceps jerk (left and right)   ☐   ☐   ☐

   Triceps jerk (left and right)   ☐   ☐   ☐

   Supinator jerk (left and right)   ☐   ☐   ☐

12 Ensures patient's comfort and dignity
   throughout; thanks patient on completion
   of examination   ☐   ☐   ☐

13 Presents findings in a fluent, logical
   manner   ☐   ☐   ☐

14 Provides a reasonable differential
   diagnosis – including pattern of weakness,
   eg UMN vs LMN; proximal vs distal   ☐   ☐   ☐

Answers

STATION 2.10

Assessment	Good	Adequate	Poor/not done
1 Appropriate introduction (full name and role)	☐	☐	☐
2 Explains purpose of examination and gains verbal consent	☐	☐	☐
3 Candidate washes their hands using the alcohol handwash provided (no marks if candidate only expresses the need to wash if handwash is provided)	☐	☐	☐
4 Observes patient from the end of the bed commenting on the presence/absence of			
Wasting of limbs		☐	☐
Fasciculation		☐	☐
Signs of stroke and other neurological disease		☐	☐
Cranial nerve lesions		☐	☐
5 Returns to the bedside and reassesses 'bulk' of the lower limbs – commenting on presence/absence of wasting/fasciculation	☐	☐	☐
6 Makes an appropriate assessment of the tone in the lower limbs	☐	☐	☐
7 Assesses the power of:			
Hip flexion		☐	☐
Hip extension		☐	☐
Knee flexion		☐	☐
Knee extension		☐	☐
Ankle dorsiflexion		☐	☐
Ankle plantar flexion		☐	☐
Foot inversion		☐	☐
Foot eversion		☐	☐

8 In all muscle groups, uses appropriate
   technique and always compares one side
   with the other.   ☐   ☐   ☐

9 Attempts to assess co-ordination   ☐   ☐   ☐

10 Makes an appropriate assessment of the
   lower limb reflexes – using appropriate
   technique and comparing right and left   ☐   ☐   ☐

11 Assesses:

   Patellar jerk (left and right)   ☐   ☐

   Ankle jerk (left and right)   ☐   ☐   ☐

12 Makes appropriate assessment of the
   plantar responses – using orange stick or
   similar   ☐   ☐   ☐

13 Asks to assess the gait of the patient

(Examiner stops the candidate – 'Please continue')

14 Ensures patient's comfort and dignity
   throughout; thanks patient on completion
   of examination   ☐   ☐   ☐

15 Presents findings in a fluent, logical
   manner   ☐   ☐   ☐

16 Provides a reasonable differential
   diagnosis – including pattern of weakness
   eg UMN vs LMN   ☐   ☐   ☐

Answers

STATION 2.11

Assessment	Good	Adequate	Poor/not done
1 Appropriate introduction (full name and role)	☐	☐	☐
2 Explains purpose of examination and gains verbal consent	☐	☐	☐
3 Candidate washes their hands using the alcohol handwash provided (no marks if candidate only expresses the need to wash if handwash is provided)	☐	☐	☐
4 Observes patient from end of the bed commenting on the presence/absence of:			
Neuropathic ulcers/burns and trauma	☐	☐	☐
Signs of neurological disease – hemiparesis; wasting; cranial nerve lesions	☐	☐	☐
Evidence of disorders associated with sensory neuropathy eg:			
• *BM stix, BM chart, insulin pens*		☐	☐
• *Signs of chronic liver disease*		☐	☐
• *Drug chart*		☐	☐
• *Anaemia (B$_{12}$ deficiency)*		☐	☐
• *Thyroid status*		☐	☐
5 Assesses light touch using cotton wool:			
Teases out piece of cotton wool		☐	☐
Explains procedure correctly		☐	☐
Tests 'normal' skin at sternal notch		☐	☐
Asks patient to close their eyes		☐	☐
Tests dermatomes of upper limbs – left and right	☐	☐	☐
Dabs (doesn't stroke) cotton wool		☐	☐

Demonstrates 'glove' distribution of
sensory loss ☐ ☐

Attempts to assess pin prick ☐ ☐

Examiner stops student – 'please continue'

6 Assesses vibration sense using tuning fork:

Explains the procedure correctly ☐ ☐

Tests 'normal skin' at sternal notch ☐ ☐

Requests patient to close their eyes ☐ ☐

Places tuning fork on interphalangeal joint
of thumb and assesses vibration sense
left and right ☐ ☐ ☐

Reassesses vibration sense at MCP joint
of thumb left and right ☐ ☐ ☐

Reassesses vibration sense at wrist, left
and right ☐ ☐ ☐

7 Assesses joint position sense (JPS)/
proprioception:

Explains procedure correctly ☐ ☐ ☐

With patient's eyes open demonstrates
movement at interphalangeal joint of
thumb (ie up and down) ☐ ☐ ☐

Asks if patient can tell the difference.
If 'no' repeats procedure proximally
at MCP joint, wrist, then elbow ☐ ☐ ☐

If 'yes' – requests patient to close eyes
and repeats procedure ☐ ☐ ☐

8 Ensures patient comfort throughout and
thanks patient on completion of
examination ☐ ☐ ☐

9 Presents findings in a fluent, logical
manner ☐ ☐ ☐

10 Provides an appropriate differential
diagnosis and causes ☐ ☐ ☐

STATION 2.12

Assessment	Good	Adequate	Poor/not done
1 Appropriate introduction (full name and role)	☐	☐	☐
2 Explains purpose of examination and gains verbal consent	☐	☐	☐
3 Candidate washes their hands using the alcohol handwash provided (no marks if candidate only expresses the need to wash if handwash is provided)	☐	☐	☐
4 Observes patient from end of the bed commenting on the presence/absence of:			
Neuropathic ulcers/burns and trauma	☐	☐	☐
Signs of neurological disease – hemiparesis, wasting, cranial nerve lesions	☐	☐	☐
Evidence of disorders associated with sensory neuropathy eg BM stix, BM chart, insulin pen	☐	☐	☐
Signs of chronic liver disease; Drug chart, anaemia (B_{12} deficiency)	☐	☐	☐
Thyroid status	☐	☐	☐
5 Assesses light touch using cotton wool:			
Teases out piece of cotton wool		☐	☐
Explains procedure correctly		☐	☐
Tests 'normal' skin at sternal notch		☐	☐
Asks patient to close their eyes		☐	☐
Tests dermatomes of lower limbs – left and right	☐	☐	☐
Dabs (doesn't stroke) cotton wool		☐	☐
Demonstrates 'stocking' distribution of sensory loss		☐	☐

6 Attempts to assess pin prick ☐ ☐ ☐

Examiner stops student – 'please continue'

7 Assesses vibration sense using tuning fork:

Explains the procedure correctly ☐ ☐ ☐

Tests 'normal skin' at sternal notch ☐ ☐

Requests patient to close their eyes ☐ ☐

Places tuning fork on interphalangeal
joint of big toe ☐ ☐

Reassesses vibration sense at MTP joint
of big toe left and right ☐ ☐ ☐

Reassesses vibration sense at medial
malleolus left and right ☐ ☐ ☐

8 Assesses joint position sense (JPS)

Explains procedure correctly ☐ ☐ ☐

With patient's eyes open demonstrates
movements of interphalangeal joint of big
toe ie up and down ☐ ☐ ☐

Asks if patient can tell the difference if
'no' – reassesses at MTP joint and ankle ☐ ☐ ☐

If 'yes' – requests patient to close their
eyes then repeats procedure ☐ ☐ ☐

9 Ensures patient comfort throughout and
thanks patient on completion of
examination ☐ ☐ ☐

10 Presents findings in a fluent, logical
manner ☐ ☐ ☐

11 Provides an appropriate differential
diagnosis and causes ☐ ☐ ☐

Answers

STATION 2.13

Assessment	Good	Adequate	Poor/not done
1 Appropriate introduction (full name and role)	☐	☐	☐
2 Explains procedure and gains verbal consent	☐	☐	☐
3 Stands at the end of the bed and observes the patient's lower limbs commenting on the presence/absence of:			
Wasting and fasciculation	☐	☐	☐
Signs of stroke and other neurological disease	☐	☐	☐
Indwelling urinary catheter		☐	☐
4 Returns to the bedside and re-assesses bulk of the lower limbs; comments on the presence/absence of fasciculation	☐	☐	☐
5 Makes an appropriate assessment of the tone in the lower limbs	☐	☐	☐
6 Assesses the power of:			
Hip flexion		☐	☐
Hip extension		☐	☐
Knee flexion		☐	☐
Knee extension		☐	☐
Ankle dorsification		☐	☐
Ankle plantar flexion		☐	☐
Foot inversion		☐	☐
Foot eversion		☐	☐
7 In all muscle groups – uses appropriate technique and always compares one side with the other	☐	☐	☐
8 Attempts to assess co-ordination		☐	☐

Examiner stops student – 'please continue'

9 Makes an appropriate assessment of the lower limb reflexes – using appropriate technique and comparing right and left ☐   ☐   ☐

10 Assesses:

   Patellar jerk (left and right) ☐   ☐   ☐

   Ankle jerk (left and right) ☐   ☐   ☐

11 Makes appropriate assessment of the plantar responses – using orange stick or similar implement ☐   ☐   ☐

12 Assesses light touch using cotton wool:

   Teases out piece of cotton wool   ☐   ☐

   Explains procedure correctly ☐   ☐   ☐

   Tests 'normal' skin at sternal notch   ☐   ☐

   Asks patient to close their eyes   ☐   ☐

   Tests dermatomes of lower limbs – left and right ☐   ☐   ☐

   Dabs (doesn't stroke) cotton wool   ☐   ☐

   Correctly defines sensory level at T10 ☐   ☐   ☐

13 Attempts to assess pin prick   ☐   ☐

Examiner stops student – 'please continue'

14 Assesses sense of vibration using tuning fork:

   Explains the procedure correctly ☐   ☐   ☐

   Tests 'normal skin' at sternal notch   ☐   ☐

   Requests patient to close their eyes   ☐   ☐

   Places tuning fork on interphalangeal joint of big toe   ☐   ☐

   Re-assesses vibration sense at MTP joint of big toe left and right ☐   ☐   ☐

   Re-assesses vibration sense at medial malleolus, tibial tuberosity and ASIS (left and right) ☐   ☐   ☐

Answers

15 Assesses joint position sense (JPS)/
    proprioception:

    Explains procedure correctly ☐ ☐ ☐

    With patient eyes open demonstrates
    movements of interphalangeal joint of
    big toe ie up and down ☐ ☐ ☐

    Asks if patient can tell the difference if
    NO – reassesses at MTP joint; then
    ankle; then knee ☐ ☐ ☐

16 Ensures patient comfort throughout and
    thanks patient on completion of
    examination ☐ ☐ ☐

17 Presents findings in a fluent, logical
    manner ☐ ☐ ☐

18 Correctly identifies spastic paraparesis
    with sensory level ☐ ☐ ☐

19 Examiner asks 'What one investigation
    would you consider as a matter of
    urgency?' (answer MRI scan of thoracic
    spine) ☐ ☐ ☐

STATION 2.14

Assessment	Good	Adequate	Poor/not done
1 Appropriate introduction (full name and role)	☐	☐	☐
2 Explains examination and gains verbal consent	☐	☐	☐
3 Candidate washes their hands using the alcohol handwash provided (no marks if candidate only expresses the need to wash if handwash is provided)	☐	☐	☐
4 Observes patient from end of the bed – commenting on presence/absence of:			
Signs of stroke disease		☐	☐
Truncal ataxia		☐	☐
Other neurological deficit eg cranial nerve lesions		☐	☐
5 Returns to the bedside – assesses for past pointing:			
Explains procedure correctly	☐	☐	☐
Examines left and right hand	☐	☐	☐
Uses appropriate technique eg distance of hand from patient	☐	☐	☐
6 Assesses for dysdiadochokinesia:			
Explains procedure correctly	☐	☐	☐
Examines left and right hand	☐	☐	☐
7 Comments on need to assess for hypotonia and hyporeflexia		☐	☐

Examiner stops student – 'please continue'

8 Assesses for nystagmus			
Explains procedure correctly	☐	☐	☐
Examines eyes to left and right gaze	☐	☐	☐

Answers

9 Assesses for cerebellar speech   ☐   ☐
   **Examiner asks 'Do you think
   they have cerebellar speech?
   What are the characteristic
   features?' (only if assessed)**   ☐   ☐   ☐

10 Assesses for cerebellar/ataxic gait   ☐   ☐   ☐

11 Maintains patient dignity throughout
   thanks patient on completion of
   examination   ☐   ☐   ☐

12 Presents findings in a fluent, logical
   manner   ☐   ☐   ☐

13 Correctly identifies unilateral/bilateral
   cerebellar signs   ☐   ☐   ☐

14 Examiner asks 'What are the common
   causes of:

   Unilateral signs?   ☐   ☐   ☐

   Bilateral signs, in a person of this age? ☐   ☐   ☐

STATION 2.15

Assessment	Good	Adequate	Poor/not done
1 Appropriate introduction (full name and role)	☐	☐	☐
2 Explains examination and gains verbal consent	☐	☐	☐
3 Observes patient – commenting on presence/absence of:			
Ptosis		☐	☐
Exophthalmos/endophthalmos		☐	☐
Divergent/convergent squint		☐	☐
Papillary asymmetry/abnormality		☐	☐
Other eye signs – red eye, periorbital signs, cataracts	☐	☐	☐
Signs of stroke and other neurological disease	☐	☐	☐
4 Tests for visual acuity:			
Explains procedure correctly	☐	☐	☐
Assesses right and left eye separately	☐	☐	☐
Defines reading, counting fingers, finger movement or perception of light – as appropriate	☐	☐	☐
5 Tests visual fields:			
Explains procedure correctly	☐	☐	☐
Assesses right and left eye separately	☐	☐	☐
Uses appropriate technique		☐	☐
Assesses all four quadrants – both eyes	☐	☐	☐
Assesses visual inattention		☐	☐

6 Tests for extraocular muscles (EOM)

Explains procedure correctly ☐ ☐ ☐

Fixes forehead of patient with free hand ☐ ☐

Moves finger in 'H' shape – observing movements of both eyes ☐ ☐ ☐

Asks patient whether they have double vision (diplopia) at all points on the 'H' ☐ ☐

Specifically looks for and comments on presence/absence of nystagmus ☐ ☐ ☐

7 Tests/assesses the pupils:

Comments on size and shape ☐ ☐ ☐

Comments on symmetry ☐ ☐

Correctly assesses direct and consensual light responses ☐ ☐ ☐

Correctly assesses accommodation, commenting on both convergence and constriction of pupils ☐ ☐ ☐

8 Attempts to perform ophthalmoscopy – **Examiner stops candidate and asks them 'What would you expect to find on ophthalmoscopy?' – or 'why would you like to perform ophthalmoscopy? Only correct/acceptable answers should score 'good'** ☐ ☐ ☐

9 Maintains patient dignity/treats patient courteously throughout, thanks patient on completion of examination ☐ ☐ ☐

10 Presents findings in a fluent logical manner ☐ ☐ ☐

11 Provides an appropriate differential diagnosis and causes ☐ ☐ ☐

STATION 2.16

Assessment	Good	Adequate	Poor/not done
1 Appropriate introduction (full name and role)	☐	☐	☐
2 Explains procedure and gains verbal consent	☐	☐	☐
3 Candidate washes their hands using the alcohol handwash provided (no marks if candidate only expresses the need to wash if handwash is provided)	☐	☐	☐
4 Observes patient, commenting on presence/absence of:			
Signs of stroke disease		☐	☐
Eye signs eg ptosis, pupillary abnormalities, cataracts	☐	☐	☐
Signs of other neurological disease		☐	☐
5 Tests for visual fields:			
Explains procedure correctly	☐	☐	☐
Assesses right and left eye separately	☐	☐	☐
Uses appropriate technique	☐	☐	☐
Assesses all four quadrants – both eyes	☐	☐	☐
6 Treats the patient courteously throughout and thanks the patient on completion of examination	☐	☐	☐
7 Presents findings in a fluent, logical manner	☐	☐	☐

8 **Examiner now shows student diagram of visual pathway – 'Please could you show me where you think the lesion is':**

Unilateral eye signs – anterior to chiasma ☐ ☐ ☐

Bitemporal hemianopia – at the chiasma ☐ ☐ ☐

Bilateral, homonymous eye signs – posterior to chiasma ☐ ☐ ☐

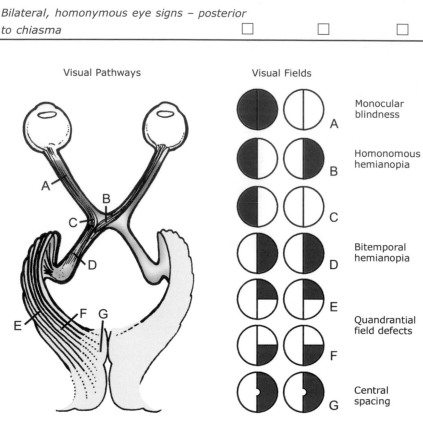

Visual Pathways   Visual Fields

A   Monocular blindness

B   Homonomous hemianopia

C

D   Bitemporal hemianopia

E   Quandrantial field defects

F

G   Central spacing

STATION 2.17

Assessment	Good	Adequate	Poor/not done
1 Appropriate introduction (full name and role)	☐	☐	☐
2 Explains examination and gains verbal consent	☐	☐	☐
3 Observes patient and comments on presence/absence of:			
Signs of stroke disease		☐	☐
Obvious cranial nerve lesions eg VII nerve palsy		☐	☐
Signs of other neurological disease eg MND or MS (in appropriately aged patients)		☐	☐
4 Returns to the bedside/chairside and assesses trigeminal nerve:			
Motor function – assessing temporalis, pterygoids and masseters, mandibular movements	☐	☐	☐
Sensory function (light touch only):			
• *Explains procedure correctly*	☐	☐	☐
• *Uses appropriate technique*	☐	☐	☐
• *Examines left and right comparing the two sides of the face*	☐	☐	☐
• **Examiner asks – 'to which nucleus do light touch signals go?'** *(answer pontine; pain and temperature have a cervical nucleus)*	☐	☐	☐
c *Attempts to do corneal reflex – examiner asks the candidate to explain procedure without allowing them to do it on patient*	☐	☐	☐

5 Assesses facial nerve motor function

- 'Give me a smile' – comments on
  symmetry   ☐   ☐   ☐

- 'Blow out your cheeks' – tests power   ☐   ☐   ☐

- 'Close your eyes tightly' – tests power ☐   ☐   ☐

- 'Look up to the ceiling/furrow your brow'
  comments on symmetry   ☐   ☐   ☐

**Sensory function – only if candidate mentions need to assess, examiner
intervenes 'what it the sensory supply of VII nerve?'**
(answer – taste to the anterior two-thirds of the tongue)   ☐   ☐

6 Assesses vestibulocochlear function

Correctly explains procedure   ☐   ☐   ☐

Performs Weber's test   ☐   ☐   ☐

Comments on normal/abnormal
response   ☐   ☐   ☐

Performs Rinne's test on left and right
ear   ☐   ☐   ☐

Comments on responses   ☐   ☐   ☐

7 Assesses glossopharyngeal/vagus function:

Asks patient to open mouth and say
'aaagh' – comments on symmetry of
palatal/uvular movement   ☐   ☐   ☐

Asks patient to say 'ecg' or 'rug' –
comments on normal/abnormal palatal
movement   ☐   ☐   ☐

**Examiner asks – 'Please show me how
you would assess their swallow mechanism**
Candidate correctly identifies:

- Patient must be sitting upright, fully
  conscious and able to understand
  commands   ☐   ☐   ☐

- Asks patient to take a sip of water and to
  hold it in their mouth   ☐   ☐   ☐

- Asks patient to swallow – commenting on presence/absence of coughing/choking ☐ ☐ ☐

- Asks patient to say eg name and address. Comments on presence/absence of 'wet voice' ☐ ☐ ☐

8 Assesses accessory function:

Asks patient to shrug shoulders and observes then tests power in left and right trapezius ☐ ☐ ☐

Tests power and bulk of left and right sternocleidomastoid ☐ ☐ ☐

9 Assesses hypoglossal function:

Observes and comments on presence/ absence of wasting and fasciculation ☐ ☐ ☐

Asks patient to stick tongue out to the right and left. Comments on normal/ abnormal response ☐ ☐ ☐

10 Treats patient courteously throughout. Thanks patient on completion of examination ☐ ☐ ☐

11 Presents findings in a fluent, logical manner ☐ ☐ ☐

12 Examiner asks:

'Could you tell me which are the cranial nerves in the "bulb"?' (answer IX–XII: medullary or bulbar nuclei) ☐ ☐ ☐

'What are the causes of a pseudobulbar palsy?' (answer – bilateral cortical lesions most commonly stroke disease multi-infarct disease, motor neurone disease) ☐ ☐ ☐

Answers

STATION 2.18

Assessment	Good	Adequate	Poor/not done
1 Appropriate introduction (full name and role)	☐	☐	☐
2 Explains examination, notes/comments on comprehension of patient	☐	☐	☐
3 Candidate washes their hands using the alcohol handwash provided (no marks if candidate only expresses the need to wash if handwash is provided)			
4 Observes patient and comments on presence/absence of:			
Signs of stroke disease		☐	☐
Cranial nerve lesions, eg VII nerve, ptosis		☐	☐
Other neurological disease		☐	☐
5 Formally assesses comprehension, ie receptive dysphasia/aphasia using 1-2-3 stage commands	☐	☐	☐
6 Formally assesses expressive dysphasia/ aphasia			
Tell me your name and address		☐	☐
Tests word finding, eg 'what is this?' (shows watch or pen)		☐	☐
Tests fluency of speech – 'tell me what you had for breakfast' (or similar)		☐	☐
7 Formally assesses dysarthria			
'Say K or G for me' – (tests palatal movement)		☐	☐
'Say M for me' – (tests facial movements)		☐	☐
'Say L for me' – (tests tongue movements)		☐	☐

8 Comments on presence/absence of dysphonia ☐ ☐

9 **Examiner asks 'What factors about the patient might stop you assessing their swallow?' Answer – drowsiness/ unconsciousness, receptive/language problems, unable to sit upright** ☐ ☐ ☐

10 Asks patient to take a sip of water and hold it in their mouth ☐ ☐ ☐

11 Asks patient to swallow water while observing and commenting on swallow mechanism ☐ ☐ ☐

12 Asks patient to say name and address commenting on presence/absence of 'wet voice' ☐ ☐ ☐

13 Comments on presence/absence of coughing or choking ☐ ☐ ☐

14 Correctly identifies patient is/is not safe to eat and drink ☐ ☐ ☐

15 **Examiner asks 'What would you recommend to the nursing staff?'** – candidate correctly recommends to remain nil by mouth or to eat and drink, observing for choking/ coughing ☐ ☐ ☐

16 Treats patient courteously throughout. Thanks patient on completion of examination ☐ ☐ ☐

17 Presents findings in a fluent, logical manner ☐ ☐ ☐

Answers

STATION 2.19

1 (C) (d)

This man has developed secondary polycythaemia due to his chronic airways disease with resultant pulmonary hypertension. The polycythaemia causes a procoagulant state which in severe cases leads to thromboembolic disease. Treatment should include treatment of the underlying airways disease and regular venesection, with the aim of reducing the haematocrit (Hct) to 0.50 or less.

2 (E) (c)

This patient demonstrates a pancytopenia secondary to an aplastic anaemia. Thrombocytopenia of less than $10 \times 10^9/l$ carries a significant risk of spontaneous bleeding, in this case a spontaneous intracranial haemorrhage. Causes of aplastic anaemia include:

- **Congenital**
  Fanconi's anaemia
- **Acquired**
  Idiopathic
  Infection – TB, hepatitis A
  Toxins – chemicals and insecticides; irradiation
  Drugs:
  > antibiotics
  > anti-epileptics
  > anti-inflammatories
  > antihistamines
  > antithyroid
  > oral hypoglycaemics
  > chemotherapeutic agents

3 (D) (e)

Primary thrombocythaemia is a relatively uncommon haematological disorder which presents with bleeding (due to abnormal platelet function), bruising and thromboembolic phenomena. It is intimately related to the myeloproliferative disorders, in particular polycythaemia rubra vera.

4 (A) (b)

Alcohol excess is shown in the peripheral blood film by macrocytosis and thrombocytopenia. Alcohol abusers are at increased risk of subdural haemorrhage because of increased falls, thrombocytopenia and coagulopathy (causing a raised INR and prolonged APTT) due to the liver's inability to produce clotting factors.

5 (B) (a)
This patient has suffered an intracranial haemorrhage due to a grossly elevated INR. This has arisen due to the interaction of erythromycin with warfarin. Caution must be used when prescribing medications for patients on oral anticoagulants and the oral contraceptive pill. (**Warfarin is an acronym made up of Wisconsin Alumni Research FoundationcoumARIN.**)

STATION 2.20

1 **(D) (e)**
2 **(E) (d)**
3 **(F) (a)**
4 **(A) (f)**
5 **(C) (b)**
6 **(B) (c)**

STATION 2.21

Sample A:Tuberculosis meningitis (TBM)
Sample B:Viral meningitis
Sample C:Bacterial meningitis

1 (A) (C)
Patients with TBM and meningococcal meningitis need all close contacts to be traced, so they may be given prophylactic treatment or screening.

2 (A) (C)
Prior to a definitive microbiological diagnosis being made, clinical features or the appearance of the CSF may demand that empirical antibiotic treatment be started. Particularly in patients where a diagnosis of streptococcal or meningococcal meningitis is suspected, any delays in confirming the diagnosis may be fatal.

3 (A) (B) (C)
All patients with suspected meningitis should be nursed in a quiet, darkened room. They often require intravenous fluids and anti-emetic therapy.

4 (C)
Neisseria meningitidis is most commonly associated with DIC but most severe bacterial meningitides may present with multi-organ failure and DIC.

5 (A)

Tuberculosis is more common in the Indian subcontinent but all the meningitides may present in this racial group.

6 (C)

The anti-streptolysin O titre (ASOT) is a marker of streptococcal infection.

7 (A) (C)

Although there may be significant changes in viral pneumonias, these are rare and the most florid changes occur with tuberculosis and bacterial infections.

8 (A) (C)

Hydrocephalus is a relatively rare complication of bacterial meningitis and TBM.

9 (A) (B)

Bacterial infections are commonly demonstrated by Gram staining; tuberculosis is demonstrated by Ziehl–Neelsen staining; viral infections are demonstrated using viral titres, electronmicroscopy and polymerase chain reaction studies; fungal infections are demonstrated using Indian ink stains.

10 (A) (B) (C)

Kernig's sign demonstrates meningeal irritation. The sign is elicited by dorsiflexing the foot which will cause pain in the spine, neck and head if positive. All the meningitides may cause a positive Kernig's sign. It may be inappropriate to perform this test in extremely ill patients.

STATION 2.22

1 (F) (d)
Oligoclonal bands, shown by protein electrophoresis, are present in the CSF in over 80% of cases of multiple sclerosis. They are formed by IgG within the CSF but the antigen they are directed against as yet remains unclear. Oligoclonal bands may also be found in the CSF of patients with sarcoidosis, SLE, Behçet's disease, neurosyphilis and viral encephalitis.

2 (D) (f)
This neonate has *Haemophilus influenzae* meningitis, which is more common in this age group. As with other bacterial meningitides there is a high protein content and a low glucose concentration. A Gram stain gives the microbiological diagnosis.

3 (E) (a)
This history is highly suggestive of meningococcal meningitis with secondary DIC. The patient should be treated empirically with high doses of benzylpenicillin and contact tracing should be arranged. All close contacts should receive prophylactic treatment with rifampicin.

4 (A) (e)
This patient gives a classical history of a subdural haemorrhage, but over 50% of patients give no history of trauma. Subdural haemorrhages are usually represented by a hyperdense concave rim around the cerebrum on CT head scan. However at 10 days they appear as an isodense rim and therefore may be overlooked.

5 (B) (c)
A sudden severe headache with an associated decreased level of consciousness must be treated as a subarachnoid haemorrhage until proven otherwise. The CSF samples are blood stained in the first 24 to 48 h but samples taken 48 to 72 h after the onset of symptoms appear discoloured due to altered blood, termed xanthochromia.

6 (C) (b)
Patients presenting with insidious worsening of a dementing type illness should have a dementia screen to exclude treatable causes. This should include VDRL, TPHA and TPA, TFTs and B12. If syphilis serology is positive the patient should have a lumbar puncture to exclude tertiary syphilis. As in this case, the patient should receive a course of benzylpenicillin after 24 h cover with steroids. This is to reduce the risk of a Jarisch–Herxheimer reaction.

STATION 2.23

fig 2.23a

(A) Parietal bone
(B) Frontal bone

(C) Supraorbital ridge
(D) Zygomatic bone
(E) Infraorbital plate of maxilla
(F) Nasal septum
(G) Mandible

fig 2.23b

(A) Parietal bone
(B) Union of sphenoid and temporal bones at pterion
(C) Pituitary fossa
(D) Petrous temporal bone
(E) Occipital bone
(F) Maxillary air sinus
(G) Mandible

STATION 2.24

1 (a) **True**   (b) **True**   (c) **True**   (d) **True**   (e) **True**

The skull X-ray shows evidence of intracranial calcification within the right cerebral hemisphere. In this case it is due to Sturge–Weber syndrome. Common causes include:

Intracranial tumours

- Benign – meningioma, pinealoma, neuroma, papilloma, craniopharyngioma, chordoma
- Malignant – oligodendroglioma, metastases

Infection

- Tuberculosis, toxoplasmosis, abscess, hydatid disease, CMV
- Basal meningitis
- Cysticercosis (infestation with tapeworm larvae)

Vascular

- Aneurysm, angioma, atherosclerosis, Sturge–Weber syndrome
- Old infarction, haematoma

Others

- Tuberose sclerosis, hypoparathyroidism, chronic renal failure.
- Toxins, lead and carbon monoxide

2 (a) **False**   (b) **False**   (c) **False**   (d) **True**   (e) **True**

This AP skull X-ray shows a compound, depressed left-sided parietal fracture. The patient had been involved in a fight and had been hit over the head with a snooker cue. This type of fracture requires surgical elevation.

3 (a) **True**   (b) **False**   (c) **False**   (d) **True**   (e) **True**

This lateral skull X-ray shows multiple lytic lesions consistent with a 'pepperpot' skull of multiple myeloma. The patient may also have an ESR > 100, paraproteinaemia, hypercalcaemia and Bence–Jones protein (light chains) in the urine. Other associations include renal failure, amyloidosis (which may be responsible for the renal failure), hyperviscocity and symptoms of pancytopenia.

STATION 2.25

fig 2.25a

(A) Right eye
(B) Left optic nerve
(C) Nasal septum
(D) Zygomatic arch
(E) Temporal lobe
(F) Sphenoidal air sinus
(G) Occipital bone
(H) Scalp
(I) Left cerebellar hemisphere
(J) Left external auditory meatus

fig 2.25b

(A) Frontal bone
(B) Falx cerebri
(C) Cerebral sulcus
(D) Cerebral gyrus
(E) Anterior horn of lateral ventricle
(F) Septum pellucidum
(G) Choroid plexus
(H) Posterior horn of lateral ventricle
(I) Occipital lobe
(J) Occipital bone

Answers

STATION 2.26

1 (a) **False**　　(b) **False**　　(c) **True**　　(d) **False**　　(e) **True**
This CT head scan shows a large left-sided frontal subdural haemaotoma. The blood has caused midline shift and obscuration of the left lateral ventricular system. There is no obstruction or hydrocephalus of the contralateral ventricular system. This disorder commonly arises due to trauma, particularly falls, although over 50% of patients with subdural haemorrhage give no such history. It is common in the elderly and in alcohol abusers. Classically, subdurals are represented by a hyperdense concave rim around the brain, as seen in this scan. However, they may be missed if the scan is taken around the tenth day after the initial haemorrhage, as during this period they may appear isodense with the grey matter, which makes them more difficult to define. Extradural haemorrhages classically form a convex interface with the grey matter.

2 (a) **True**　　(b) **False**　　(c) **True**　　(d) **False**　　(e) **True**
This CT scan shows intraventricular blood caused by a large subarachnoid haemorrhage. The headache is classically sudden and severe in nature and is associated with a depressed level of consciousness. Patients require supportive therapy with fluids and should be given nimodipine. Patients with a depressed level of consciousness should be electively intubated and ventilated, this helps by reducing intracranial pressure. Neurosurgery should be considered but may not be appropriate in all cases.

3 (a) **False**　　(b) **True**　　(c) **False**　　(d) **False**　　(e) **True**
The third scan shows a large right frontal infarct. There is no midline shift or obscuration of the ventricles. Patients with large cerebral infarcts are likely to be hypertensive prior to their stroke, as this is the principal risk factor, and are often hypertensive on admission because of the vascular response to the ischaemic insult. The treatment of the associated hypertension is still unclear and at present hypertension is not treated for 48 to 72 h post stroke. This may change as thrombolytic therapy in stroke becomes more common practice. All patients should be considered for formal anticoagulation with warfarin, or secondary prophylaxis with aspirin and/or dipyridamole slow-release therapy.

STATION 2.27

1 (a) **False**   (b) **False**   (c) **False**   (d) **False**   (e) **False**

This CT head scan shows a large intracerebral bleed within the right cerebral hemisphere. Blood appears white on a scan and should not be confused with contrast. There is no evidence of midline shift or hydrocephalus which may occur with such a large bleed. This patient presented with a GCS of 3 which never improved and he died 24 h after admission. It is important to perform a scan in order to exclude treatable causes of a depressed level of consciousness, and to institute appropriate care, which may include withdrawing 'active' treatment and keeping the patient palliated until death.

2 (a) **False**   (b) **True**   (c) **False**   (d) **False**   (e) **True**

This contrast-enhanced CT head scan shows an enhancing lesion in the right occipital area, its appearance being consistent with a meningioma. The patient will not be blind, but will have a left homonymous field defect. The tumour should be excised neurosurgically and if proven to be a malignant meningioma by histology, postoperative radiotherapy should be offered to the patient.

3 (a) **True**   (b) **False**   (c) **True**   (d) **True**   (e) **False**

The first contrast-enhanced CT head scan shows evidence of a ring enhancing lesion with surrounding oedema in the left frontal area. Further views show multiple similar lesions consistent with multiple metastases. The differential cause of a ring enhancing lesion include a cerebral abscess, for example toxoplasmosis, aspergillus and bacterial emboli associated with endocarditis, and malignancy such as cerebral metastases and lymphoma.

STATION 2.28a

Patient history

I am a 23-year-old fashion model who was diagnosed as having epilepsy six months ago. Since diagnosis I have made no changes to my very hectic life and as a consequence the fits have become increasingly more frequent and severe. In the last two weeks I have had several fits, the last at a big fashion show in Milan. It was after this episode that my agent refused to book me for any more work until I get sorted out. I drink 20–30 units of alcohol per week, mainly in the form of white wine. Occasionally I do drink a lot more at parties. I smoke 10 to 20 cigarettes per day and use occasional recreational drugs including cannabis and cocaine. I am taking no medications other than the oral contraceptive pill and am still driving a car on a regular basis. No one has ever explained the diagnosis or the precipitating factors of my problems. I am very keen to make lifestyle changes but am very reluctant to start medical treatment. I am very upset about having epilepsy in case people think I have a psychiatric problem. I am also worried about the consequences for my career and lifestyle.

Assessment	Good	Adequate	Poor/not done
1 Appropriate introduction (full name and role)	☐	☐	☐
2 Explains the purpose of the interview	☐	☐	☐
3 Establishes the present level of patient understanding about the diagnosis, complications and treatment	☐	☐	☐
4 Establishes patient understanding of precipitating factors such as alcohol, recreational drugs and flashing lights (relevant to job)	☐	☐	☐
5 Discusses the need to stop/avoid precipitating factors	☐	☐	☐
6 Discusses the issue of driving – must register with DVLC; can resume driving if fit-free for one year	☐	☐	☐
7 Discusses the possibility of avoiding drug therapy if precipitating factors are stopped/avoided	☐	☐	☐

8 Discusses the reasons for and against
   starting drug therapy:

   Will still have to change lifestyle   ☐   ☐

   Will have to take medications regularly   ☐   ☐

   Mentions side-effects   ☐   ☐

   Mentions interactions with the OCP   ☐   ☐

   *Emphasises medications may not
   stop fits*   ☐   ☐

   *Mentions possibility of combination
   therapy*   ☐   ☐

9 Elicits patient's concerns and responds
   sensitively   ☐   ☐   ☐

10 Gives clear well-paced information   ☐   ☐   ☐

11 Checks patient's understanding of
   information   ☐   ☐   ☐

12 Systematic and organised approach   ☐   ☐   ☐

SP to mark

13 The doctor was empathic   ☐   ☐   ☐

Answers

Comment

A diagnosis of epilepsy can be quite a shock and depressing for a patient, particularly a young adult. They should be reassured that in the majority of cases a patient is fit-free and off medication within five years. There are of course a small minority of difficult, resistant cases.

Initially, if the patient has had only 1–2 fits of short duration, a probationary period may be agreed between the neurologist and the patient. Lifestyle changes, for example excluding alcohol, should be instituted in this period and the patient should be excluded from driving and operating heavy machinery. Epilepsy may stop the patient working and this may need to be discussed with a social worker. If the patient continues to have seizures then drug treatment should be instituted.

In most cases, a single agent should be chosen and this should be tailored to the individual patient, particularly if they are on other medications (eg the OCP). The patient should be advised of the possible side-effects and interactions and the regime clearly explained particularly if loading doses need to be started. Treatment and the seizures should be monitored with easy access clinics and help for the patient.

First-line therapies	Advantages	Side-effects
Sodium valproate	Drug of choice Fewer side-effects No monitoring of levels required	Acute hepatic insufficiency Hair thinning (hair grows back but may be curly!) Weight gain
Carbamazepine	Relatively few side-effects Simple to predict changes in dose as there is an almost linear relationship between oral dose and serum levels	Commonly causes a transient erythematous rash Bone marrow suppression (agranulocytosis) Nausea and vomiting Ataxia, blurred vision Cholestatic jaundice
Phenytoin	Effective in tonic–clonic seizure Drug choice in emergency treatment	Multiple side-effects Particularly 'user unfriendly' in the young adult Narrow therapeutic window

Second-line therapies	Advantages	Side-effects
Lamotrigine	Add-on therapy First-line treatment Reduces seizure in 25% of patients	May exacerbate seizures Skin rashes Sedation Hepatic dysfunction Flu-like symptoms on starting
Vigabatrin	Add-on therapy Reduction of seizure frequency in 50% of patients	Sedation Multiple neurological and behavioural problems Confusion/agitation Eye problems

Other drugs that should be considered as 'add-on therapies' include primidone, phenobarbitone, clonazepam and clobazam.

STATION 2.29

1 (C) (f)

Beta interferon remains a controversial treatment for multiple sclerosis. Studies have shown benefits of therapy in patients with relapsing disease with reduction in the frequency of acute relapses. However, there has been little proven effect on overall prognosis and disability and some health authorities within the UK have refused to endorse the drug's prescription, due to cost.

2 (D) (e)

Anticholinesterases form the mainstay of treatment in myasthenia gravis. Immunosuppressants are used in more severe disease and, as in this case, the patient may require thymectomy.

3 (E) (a)

Parkinson's disease is treated using L-dopa therapy combined with peripheral decarboxylase inhibitors. Other therapies include dopaminergic agonists such as pergolide and bromocriptine, selegiline and the recent addition of catecholamine-O-methyl transferase (COMT) inhibitors. No therapy has yet been shown to change the insidious progression of the disease.

4 (A) (c)

Anticholinesterase inhibitors have recently been shown to slow the progression of Alzheimer's disease. However, as with beta interferon and COMT inhibitors, this therapy has not been shown to change the overall prognosis and therefore its use has been restricted within the UK.

5 (F) (b)

This is a classical history of giant cell arteritis. The patient should be started on high dose steroids immediately and the diagnosis proven by temporal artery biopsy and ESR. There is a 48 h window between starting treatment and taking a biopsy, after which the diagnostic histological changes disappear.

6 (B) (d)

This is a classical triad of normal pressure hydrocephalus, urinary incontinence, confusion and gait dyspraxia. The treatment of choice is neurosurgical insertion of a ventriculo-peritoneal shunt. The title of normal pressure is a misnomer, studies having shown that such patients have fluctuating CSF pressures and that the insertion of the shunt reduces the effects of any rises that may occur.

Answers

STATION 2.30

Patient history

I am a second year medical student and was admitted two days ago with a moderately severe headache which came on insidiously over 3–4 days. The headache has been poorly relieved despite intravenous fluids and analgesia but the CT head scan performed yesterday was normal. The registrar has explained to me that I need a lumbar puncture but I am not very clear as to what this means. Everyone just assumes I understand because I'm a medic. Lumbar puncture sounds quite alarming – can the spinal cord be damaged? I'm also worried about what could be wrong and how serious it could be. I've got important exams coming up.

Assessment	Good	Adequate	Poor/not done
1 Appropriate introduction (full name and role)	☐	☐	☐
2 Explains what the interview is to be about	☐	☐	☐
3 Establishes present patient understanding of the lumbar puncture	☐	☐	☐
4 Explains the following steps of the procedure:			
Position: *Patient should be placed on the bed in the left lateral position with the knees tucked up into the chest OR sitting up leaning over the patient table which is topped with pillows*	☐	☐	☐
Patient will feel some pushing on the back and around the tops of the hips as the landmarks are mapped out	☐	☐	☐
Skin is cleaned with antiseptic, which is cold, and then the lower back is covered with surgical sheets	☐	☐	☐
Local area is then injected with local anaesthetic, which 'stings a little'	☐	☐	☐
Patient will feel some more pushing as the needle is inserted through the skin	☐	☐	☐

A small amount of fluid (3ml) is then drained from the spine and this is sent to the laboratory to be looked at under the microscope	☐	☐	☐
The patient will be expected to lie flat for 6–8 h after the procedure and will be given analgesia and fluids	☐	☐	☐
Complications: *Local pain at the puncture site and headache are the primary problems*	☐	☐	☐
5 Elicits patient's concerns and responds appropriately	☐	☐	☐
6 Invites patient questions and answers appropriately	☐	☐	☐
7 Checks patient's understanding	☐	☐	☐
8 Systematic and organised approach	☐	☐	☐

Answers

Comment

What's the definition of a lumbar puncture? Two very frightened people joined by a needle! One should always remember this joke when performing a lumbar puncture. The patient is often very ill and the thought of a doctor putting a needle into their spine makes them even more anxious. The explanation and reassurance prior to the actual procedure is therefore extremely important. The procedure is relatively simple and in experienced hands takes only a few minutes. From a practical point of view the important elements are the positioning of the patient, the drawing out of the landmarks and the insertion of the needle.

Patient position: There are two accepted ways of positioning the patient. (a) The patient is placed in the left lateral position with their lumbar spine parallel to the edge of the bed. They are manoeuvred so their back is on the edge of the bed, or (b) the patient is sat upright leaning over a support, such as the patient's table covered with pillows. Whichever position one uses, always remember to adjust the height of the bed to allow comfort and ease during the procedure.

The landmarks: The ideal interspace to use is the L4/5 space which is conveniently located by drawing a horizontal line between the iliac crests. The vertebral spines should be palpated and the space between them defined. It is important that one can confidently feel this space, otherwise the procedure will be extremely difficult. The space may be marked by using the cap of a biro pen. By pushing gently the cap impression is left in the skin. The advantage of this method is that the impression will not be removed by the antiseptic cleaning of the skin.

Insertion of the needle: Once the interspace has been infiltrated with local anaesthetic, one is ready to insert the needle. The needle should be placed at 90 degrees to the skin and inserted through the local anaesthetic needle tracks. In the correct position the needle will pass easily to the spinal ligament, and with a slight 'give' pass into the canal. On withdrawal of the introducer, clear CSF should flow back. Commonly one hits bone rather than the ligament. If this occurs, partially withdraw the needle and re-insert at a slightly different angle, using the landmarks for reference.

In acute headache only 3–4 drops of CSF need be collected in each of three sterile specimen pots. Two are sent to biochemistry for glucose and protein estimation, the third is sent to microbiology for microscopy and culture. (A simultaneous serum glucose is needed for comparison). If viral causes are suspected CSF should be collected for polymerase chain reaction (PCR) studies and viral titres. Always check with the laboratory prior to the procedure what specimens are required for a particular disorder.

STATION 2.31

Patient history

I am 43 years old and have three children. Recently, my eldest daughter, aged 14 years old was killed in a hit-and-run road traffic accident. Prior to the accident I was always quite a happy and carefree person and never thought of myself as unhappy or depressed. Since the accident three months ago, I have not been out of the house more than four or five times and have lost three stone in weight. I eat very little; surviving on a few cups of tea and occasional snacks which my husband forces me to eat. I have been unable to go back to work and have lost interest in everything around me. I sleep fitfully through the night and wake at 4.30 or 5 o'clock every morning. I can't accept my daughter's death and have thought several times about ending it all but have never made any plans to carry out any of these thoughts as I must carry on for the sake of my other children. I have no thoughts about the future. My GP placed me on some Valium after the accident but I've refused to see her again. I drink little alcohol, no more than 2–3 units a week, but I smoke 30 cigarettes per day. I have no previous history of psychiatric illness but remember my mother was treated for depression when I was a little girl. Do you think I will need to go into hospital?

Assessment	Good	Adequate	Poor/not done
1 Appropriate introduction (full name and role)	☐	☐	☐
2 Explains purpose of interview	☐	☐	☐
3 Establishes the preceding life events and duration of the presenting complaint	☐	☐	☐
4 Investigates patient's insight into her illness and reasons for attendance at the clinic	☐	☐	☐
5 Asks about specific symptoms of depression:			
Early morning wakening/sleep disturbance	☐	☐	☐
Loss of appetite and weight	☐	☐	☐
Loss of energy and enthusiasm	☐	☐	☐
View of environment/future	☐	☐	☐
Self-harm/suicidal intentions	☐	☐	☐

6 Establishes family/personal history of psychiatric illness ☐ ☐ ☐

7 Establishes premorbid personality ☐ ☐ ☐

8 Establishes drug, alcohol and smoking history ☐ ☐ ☐

9 Appropriate non-verbal behaviour ☐ ☐ ☐

10 Uses an appropriate questioning technique ☐ ☐ ☐

11 Summarises history back to patient ☐ ☐ ☐

12 Makes explicit empathic statements ☐ ☐ ☐

13 Systematic, organised approach ☐ ☐ ☐

14 When asked, decides patient has reactive depression and does not need to be admitted ☐ ☐ ☐

SP to mark

15 This student helped me to talk about my feelings ☐ ☐ ☐

Management of such a patient should include bereavement counselling, antidepressants eg SSRIs, and possible psychoanalysis.

STATION 2.32

Patient history

I am 23 years old and I lost my job as an apprentice car mechanic three months ago. I have always been a bit of a loner and find it difficult to make friends easily. I have had three or four jobs over the past five years and never seem to be able to settle down to anything for a sustained period. However, I was really enjoying my job in the garage and it was a real shock that I was fired. Since then they have been telling me that the world is against me and that the reason I lost my job was because they are all jealous of me. I killed the dog because they told me that he was an evil force and would kill people very soon if I didn't kill him. My mother and father are plotting with them to keep me away from my work and that's why I had to set the house on fire.

No-one seems to believe me that they are all around and that they are going to take over the world. If they knew I was here they would try to kill me. I was found by a car park attendant at the top of the local multi-storey car park trying to climb over the railings on the top floor because they said they had given me the power to fly. They told me to throw myself off the car park and prove it to the world.

I have never seen them but know they are around. They are always talking about me, and I have heard my name several times on the television recently. I do not drink any alcohol or take recreational drugs but smoke 20 cigarettes per day. I was diagnosed as being depressed six months ago by my GP but only took the tablets for a few months. I don't know if anyone in my family has been mentally ill.

I am not aware that I have been behaving in an abnormal way.

Assessment	Good	Adequate	Poor/not done
1 Appropriate introduction (full name and role)	☐	☐	☐
2 Explains the purpose of the interview	☐	☐	☐
3 Establishes the nature and duration of the 'strange behaviour'	☐	☐	☐
4 Investigates the patient's insight into his behaviour	☐	☐	☐

Answers

5 Establishes/excludes the presence of first
rank symptoms of schizophrenia:

Thought insertion ☐ ☐

Thought broadcasting ☐ ☐

Thought withdrawal ☐ ☐

Somatic passivity ☐ ☐

Delusional perception ☐ ☐

External control of emotion ☐ ☐

6 Establishes alcohol and recreational
drug history ☐ ☐ ☐

7 Establishes/excludes thoughts of
deliberate self-harm ☐ ☐ ☐

8 Establishes personal and family history
of psychiatric illness ☐ ☐ ☐

9 Establishes/excludes precipitating
life events ☐ ☐ ☐

10 Uses appropriate non-verbal behaviour ☐ ☐ ☐

11 Uses an appropriate questioning style ☐ ☐ ☐

12 Summarises history back to patient ☐ ☐ ☐

13 Systematic, organised approach ☐ ☐ ☐

SP to mark

14 I found it easy to talk to this student ☐ ☐ ☐

15 I understood the questions ☐ ☐ ☐

Diagnosis
Acute psychosis secondary to schizophrenia.

STATION 2.33

Patient history

I am 36 years old and work as a prostitute. I recently found out that I am HIV positive. I was diagnosed only two days ago and since then have been working out how to kill myself. Tonight my flatmate told me that she was seeing her new boyfriend and would not be home till tomorrow 'if everything went to plan'. I drank a litre bottle of rum before taking 50 paracetamol tablets, 100 temazepam tablets and 50 Valium tablets which I had acquired on the street this afternoon. Before taking the tablets I wrote three letters, one to my parents, one to my little girl and one to my flatmate, telling them all I was sorry and that I couldn't face life being HIV positive. Unfortunately, I was discovered by my flatmate, who had come home unexpectedly, as her boyfriend had been called out on an emergency job and so couldn't make the date.

I have no good thoughts about the future and I will kill myself as soon as I am out of the hospital.

I took two small overdoses as a teenager, as my father was sexually abusing me. I do not know of anyone else in the family who has attempted or committed suicide. I think I am usually quite a happy-go-lucky person and have never been diagnosed as having a psychiatric illness. I am on no regular medications, I drink 30 to 40 units of alcohol per week (mainly in the form of rum and coke), and occasionally use cocaine and speed. I smoke 20 to 30 cigarettes per day and, occasionally, cannabis.

Do you think I need to be admitted to hospital? If so, why?

Assessment	Good	Adequate	Poor/not done
1 Appropriate introduction (full name and role)	☐	☐	☐
2 Explains what interview will be about	☐	☐	☐
3 Establishes events leading up to overdose	☐	☐	☐
4 Establishes timing and method of overdose	☐	☐	☐
5 Establishes suicidal intent:			
Planning		☐	☐
Place		☐	☐
Writing/content of note		☐	☐
Present view of suicide attempt		☐	☐

Answers

6 Establishes previous and family history of deliberate self-harm ☐ ☐ ☐

7 Establishes previous personal and family history of psychiatric illness ☐ ☐ ☐

8 Establishes alcohol, cigarette and recreational drug history ☐ ☐ ☐

9 Establishes premorbid personality and view of the future ☐ ☐ ☐

10 Uses appropriate non-verbal behaviour ☐ ☐ ☐

11 Uses an appropriate questioning style ☐ ☐ ☐

12 Marks explicit empathic statements ☐ ☐ ☐

13 Systematic, organised approach ☐ ☐ ☐

14 When asked indicates that patient needs to be admitted because of high suicidal risk ☐ ☐ ☐

SP to mark

15 This doctor was not judgemental ☐ ☐ ☐

Diagnosis

Serious drug overdose for which the patient needs to be admitted.

STATION 2.34

Patient history from spouse

My husband, who is 28, has been acting very strangely since he lost his job in a city accountancy firm. I am very worried about him and this is why I've come to see the doctor. My husband used to be outgoing and extrovert in nature until six months ago, when he got a promotion, which, I felt, was too much for him. Initially he handled things okay but over several months he began to drink heavily. He seemed to be working almost every night including weekends and became very snappy and withdrawn. The GP saw him, thought he was depressed, and started him on some Prozac. Things improved for a little but two months ago the company was taken over by a larger American company and redundancies were made, which included my husband. Over the last month his behaviour has become increasingly bizarre. He has run up large debts with the bank, telling the bank manager and friends that, in fact, he has been promoted to an executive position in the American company and is waiting to go to New York in the spring. He is sleeping less than 2–3 hours per night and I have started sleeping in the spare room, as he has become increasingly sexually demanding.

He seems to believe all he is saying and has no regard for me or the children. As far as I know he is not taking any recreational drugs, although he is still drinking a bottle of whisky per day. He has not been taking his antidepressant tablets and is on no other medications. He has no other significant medical or psychiatric history but I know his mother was admitted to a psychiatric hospital when we first started going out, as she had a breakdown and tried to kill herself.

I am very worried about his state of mind and about out future. I can't make any plans but we are now in financial difficulties and I have to think about our children. He is very different from the person I married.

Assessment	Good	Adequate	Poor/not done
1 Appropriate introduction (full name and role)	☐	☐	☐
2 Explains what interview will be about and gains comment	☐	☐	☐
3 Establishes duration and nature of presenting complaint	☐	☐	☐
4 Establishes premorbid events leading up to illness	☐	☐	☐

5 Establishes symptoms suggestive
   of mania:

   Increased energy ☐ ☐

   Disturbed sleep ☐ ☐

   Increased libido ☐ ☐

   Grandiose ideas ☐ ☐

   Delusional ideas. ☐ ☐

6 Establishes symptoms of depression
   and patient insight into illness ☐ ☐ ☐

7 Establishes alcohol, cigarette and
   recreational drug history ☐ ☐ ☐

8 Establishes personal and family
   history of psychiatric illness ☐ ☐ ☐

9 Establishes premorbid personality ☐ ☐ ☐

10 Elicits patient's concerns and responds
   sensitively ☐ ☐ ☐

11 Summarises history back to patient ☐ ☐ ☐

12 Makes explicit empathic statements ☐ ☐ ☐

13 Systematic, organised approach ☐ ☐ ☐

SP to mark

14 This student helped me to talk ☐ ☐ ☐

Diagnosis
Acute mania (on the background of depression) precipitated by loss of job. This man
has a bipolar disorder (ie showing symptoms of both mania and depression).

STATION 2.35

Patient history

I am 43 years old and the manager of a semi-professional football team. I need advice about an alcohol withdrawal programme.

I was brought up surrounded by alcohol; my mother and father both drank heavily, my father often becoming violent towards me when drunk. I could have been a professional footballer but my drinking problems stopped me ever progressing from the lower leagues. I have drunk excessively since I was 16 years old, mostly in the form of beer and whisky. Most days I will have a large whisky or two in my breakfast coffee and then have a few whiskies through the morning. At lunch I will have 2–3 pints of lager and a couple of whiskies and then in the evening a bottle of whisky, a few beers and occasionally a bottle of wine.

I have lost two jobs in the last five years because of my drinking, and my wife left me two years ago when I lost all our savings through drinking and gambling. I have tried to give up several times and thought I had it under control but I have never tried to dry out formally.

Two weeks ago I got the fright of my life when I was rushed to hospital after vomiting all the blood in my body and nearly dying. The doctors had to look down into my gullet several times to stop the bleeding. The consultant told me that I have severely damaged my liver and that if I don't stop drinking I will almost certainly die in the next year or two. I am determined to put my life back together again and have decided that I must stop drinking. I understand that it will be difficult but I have not had a drink for two days and, although I am a bit shaky, I think I can manage to stop this time.

Assessment	Good	Adequate	Poor/not done
1 Appropriate introduction (full name and role)	☐	☐	☐
2 Explains purpose of interview and asks for consent	☐	☐	☐
3 Establishes the duration of patient's alcohol problems	☐	☐	☐
4 Investigates patient's view of his alcohol abuse	☐	☐	☐

5 Establishes drinking patterns:

Drinking alone, drinking in the mornings,
drinking to stop symptoms of withdrawal   ☐   ☐   ☐

6 Establishes quantity of alcohol consumed
   per 24 h (divided into wine, spirits
   and beer)   ☐   ☐   ☐

7 Establishes whether the patient has tried
   to withdraw from alcohol in the past
   (formal and informal)   ☐   ☐   ☐

8 Agrees patient has good motivation and
   should be placed on the programme   ☐   ☐   ☐

9 Uses an appropriate questioning
   technique   ☐   ☐   ☐

10 Summarises the history back to the
    patient   ☐   ☐   ☐

11 Checks patient's understanding of and
    reasons for detoxification   ☐   ☐   ☐

12 Systematic, organised approach   ☐   ☐   ☐

SP to mark

13 The doctor was not judgemental   ☐   ☐   ☐

Diagnosis

Long-term alcohol abuser now highly motivated to undergo detoxification after large
GI bleed secondary to oesophageal varices.

STATION 2.36

Patient history

I am 27 years old and have always been fit and well. I have come to see you because I just can't stop washing my hands. I've always been very concerned with keeping clean and tidy but recently it has got to the point where I have to wash my hands at least 3–4 times an hour. I realise that it's absolutely mad to keep doing it but I just can't help myself. I have now made my hands bleed and they are painful and raw. I have tried to stop but have only managed a few hours and then I feel very anxious that I am getting dirty and have to start again. I have never heard voices telling me to wash my hands. Neither I nor my family have any history of psychiatric illness. There has been no recent upheaval in my life and I am otherwise well. I do not drink any alcohol, smoke cigarettes or take any recreational drugs. I work as a website designer and people are stating to comment on the number of times I go to the loo.

Assessment	Good	Adequate	Poor/not done
1 Appropriate introduction (full name and role)	☐	☐	☐
2 Explains what interview to be about and asks for consent	☐	☐	☐
3 Establishes the duration of symptoms and any precipitating life events	☐	☐	☐
4 Establishes frequency of hand washing and events which seem to precipitate the need to wash	☐	☐	☐
5 Investigates patient's insight into problem	☐	☐	☐
6 Excludes symptoms of external control and features suggestive of psychosis	☐	☐	☐
7 Excludes symptoms of depression and anxiety	☐	☐	☐
8 Excludes previous personal and family history of psychiatric illness, smoking or recreational drugs	☐	☐	☐
9 Uses an appropriate questioning technique	☐	☐	☐

Answers

	Good	Adequate	Poor/not done
10 Summarises the history back to the patient	☐	☐	☐
11 Systematic, organised approach	☐	☐	☐
SP to mark			
12 This student was empathic	☐	☐	☐

Diagnosis
Obsessive compulsive disorder.

STATION 2.37

Patient history

I am 72 years old and am usually fit and well. I was admitted five days ago with unstable angina. I have been well on the ward until this evening. I am now convinced that the nursing staff and other patients are plotting to kill me and I must be allowed to go home. I know my name, date of birth and the correct day and month and can count backwards from 20 to 1. I do not know where I am, the correct year, my age or the time of day. I can remember the objects and address at one minute but not at five minutes. I demand to go home and will not listen to any reasoning by any doctor.

Assessment	Good	Adequate	Poor/not done
1 Appropriate introduction (full name and role)	☐	☐	☐
2 Establishes patient's identity	☐	☐	☐
3 Establishes why the patient wants to go home	☐	☐	☐
4 Performs a mental test score on the patient, to include:			
Name		☐	☐
Place		☐	☐
Day		☐	☐
Month		☐	☐
Year		☐	☐
Time of day		☐	☐
Date of birth/age		☐	☐

*Address or three objects to remember
after 1 and 5 minutes* ☐ ☐

Prime minister's name ☐ ☐

Monarch ☐ ☐

Counting backwards from 20 ☐ ☐

**At this point the examiner, acting as the staff nurse
on the ward, should ask the doctor if
he/she would like to see any of the charts**

5 Asks for the observation chart to exclude
   pyrexia, changes in pulse and blood
   pressure ☐ ☐ ☐

6 Asks for the drug chart to exclude
   iatrogenic causes of confusion ☐ ☐ ☐

7 When asked realises the patient is acutely
   confused and must stay in hospital ☐ ☐ ☐

8 Reassures the patient and explains that
   she must stay in hospital ☐ ☐ ☐

9 Uses an appropriate questioning technique ☐ ☐ ☐

10 Empathic approach, non-patronising ☐ ☐ ☐

Diagnosis

Acute confusional state secondary to probable sepsis.

If the doctor asks for the patient's observations:

Pulse 120 regular, BP 110/80, temperature 39.5°C, O_2 saturation 96% on air.

Drug chart – ISMN 20 mg bd; aspirin 75 mg od; frusemide 40 mg od;
perindopril 4 mg od

Comment

When confronted with an acutely confused patient the house officer often forgets to
search for a cause and opts to sedate the patient. This is a dangerous course to choose
and should be considered only when organic causes of confusion have been excluded.

Sepsis, electrolyte derangement and iatrogenic causes such as drugs should be
considered. If sedation is necessary then small doses of haloperidol should be used.
In the younger patient up to 10 mg may be necessary but for the elderly 0.5 to 1 mg
is often enough.

STATION 2.38

1 (C) (f)
This patient presents with a history of decompensated alcoholic liver disease with resulting encephalopathy. Low Na^+ is caused by secondary hyperaldosteronism, hypoglycaemia by poor glycogen stores in diseased liver.

2 (F) (d)
Carcinoma of the lung may produce several ectopic hormones including parathyroid-like hormone, ACTH and SIADH. A high calcium may also be caused by metastatic bone disease.

3 (E) (b)
This young woman presents with a history suggestive of diabetes (polyuria and polydypsia) associated with an acute chest infection. The infection has caused her diabetes to spiral out of control leading to her hyperglycaemia and precomatose state. To prove the diagnosis of ketoacidosis, a bicarbonate and a urinary ketone level are needed but with the information available this is the most appropriate answer.

4 (A) (e)
Long-term steroid suppression of the adrenal glands is the most common cause of Addison's disease. Addisonian crisis may be precipitated in such patients when they are unable to take their steroids, for example when vomiting, or when placed under extreme stress such as in an acute, severe illness such as a myocardial infarction. In such circumstances the patient should receive intravenous hydrocortisone until such time as they are well enough to restart their tablets.

5 (B) (a)
Uraemia may cause an acute confusional state that may progress to coma. Other biochemical markers of chronic renal impairment include low bicarbonate, indicating metabolic acidosis, low calcium, and raised phosphate. Often these patients also have an anaemia of chronic disease.

6 (D) (c)
Atypical pneumonias are a common cause of the syndrome of inappropriate ADH secretion. *Legionnella* infection causes legionnaires' disease, characterised by an acute respiratory tract infection with diarrhoea and confusion. Biochemically there may be low sodium and hypophosphataemia.

STATION 2.39

1 (E) (d)
Neuroleptic malignant syndrome is a well recognised phenomenon associated with the initiation and the increase of neuroleptic drugs such as phenothiazines and butyrophenones. The syndrome is characterised by hyperpyrexia, muscle rigidity, tachycardia and impaired consciousness. Treatment should include immediate cessation of the responsible drug and symptomatic treatment with dantrolene which may ease the muscle rigidity.

2 (A) (e)
Brain tumours, including metastases, particularly in the frontal lobes may produce personality changes and aggressive behaviour. This patient may have SIADH secondary to the primary lung tumour or to the secondary brain metastases. The raised calcium may be due to parathryoid-like hormone or bony metastases.

3 (D) (a)
Manic depressives are principally treated with lithium. It has a narrow therapeutic window and commonly causes toxic side-effects. Diabetes insipidus indicated by the polyuria and the raised sodium is a recognised effect.

4 (C) (b)
This patient has several indicators that he is a long-term alcohol abuser – low urea and platelet count with a raised MCV. Alcohol withdrawal per se does not cause acute changes in indices.

5 (B) (c)
SSRIs are a relatively new group of antidepressants, they include fluoxetine, paroxetine and sertraline. Hyponatraemia is a relatively common side-effect, particularly in the elderly, and may require cessation of the drug.

Answers

STATION 2.40

1 (C) (e)

Vascular or multi-infarct dementia is often a clinical diagnosis based on a stepwise progressive dementia associated with a previous history of atherosclerotic disease and is confirmed by multiple infarcts seen on CT scan of the head. Alongside Alzheimer's disease it is responsible for 75% of all cases of dementia.

2 (E) (g)

Normal pressure hydrocephalus is diagnosed clinically by the classical triad of confusion, incontinence and gait dyspraxia. It is confirmed by CT head scan and lumbar puncture which show dilated ventricles and a normal opening pressure of 10–15 cm of CSF. Normal pressure is perhaps a misnomer as studies have shown that these patients have episodic rises in their CSF pressure, which is thought to be responsible for the confusion.

3 (A) (f)

Hypothyroidism is a reversible cause of dementia and all patients with a diagnosis of dementia should have a thyroid function test. If found to be hypothyroid, thyroxine should be introduced at a low dose of 25 µg daily for a week or two, then increased slowly over several weeks until the TSH is suppressed and the free thyroxine increased into the normal physiological range.

4 (G) (b)

Tertiary syphilis may produce a dementing-type illness associated with cranial and peripheral nerve lesions. This syndrome is known as general paralysis of the insane (GPI) and causes mixed upper and lower motor neurone signs in the lower limbs (ie areflexia and extensor plantars). Neurosyphilis is confirmed when the CSF is positive for VDRL, TPHA and FTA. It is treated with intravenous penicillin with steroid cover for 24 h prior to the antibiotics to prevent the Jarisch–Herxheimer reaction.

5 (F) (c)

This patient has B_{12} deficiency which may cause a dementing illness associated with anaemia, and sub-acute combined degeneration of the spinal cord (SACD) which causes a peripheral neuropathy associated with progressive lower limb weakness and ataxia. The patient should be treated with intramuscular B_{12} injections.

6 (D) (a)

Creutzfeldt–Jakob disease has two forms, a genetic disease and an acquired form. It presents with a rapid dementia associated with variable progressive neurological signs and symptoms. The diagnosis may be confirmed by EEG, CSF prion proteins and brain biopsy, although the latter must be undertaken in strictly controlled conditions and the instruments destroyed if the diagnosis is proved.

7 (B) (d)

Hypoparathyroidism is a relatively rare cause of dementia. It presents with hypocalcaemia which, if severe enough, causes seizures and tetany. It may produce ectopic calcification in the cornea and the central nervous system. The treatment should include intravenous calcium supplementation, if tetany is apparent, add oral 1-hydroxycholecalciferol.

STATION 2.41a

Patient history

I am 23 years old and was diagnosed with schizophrenia, diagnosed two-and-a-half years ago. After an initial period when I was quite ill and required a lot of inpatient care, I am now relatively well controlled and, after discussion with my CPN and the registrar, I would like to know more about depot injections. Although I have had several talks with the CPN I am not sure about the timing of the injections, what the injections consist of, at what sites I'll be injected and how this will improve things for me.

I'm a bit scared of needles as they remind me of when I was really sick. I am hoping to go to university and am very keen to try the treatment if I am suitable.

Assessment	Good	Adequate	Poor/not done
1 Appropriate introduction (full name and role) and asks for patient consent	☐	☐	☐
2 Establishes patient identity and reason for attending the clinic	☐	☐	☐
3 Establishes present understanding of the treatment	☐	☐	☐
4 Establishes present method of treatment and control	☐	☐	☐
5 Explains advantages of depot injections	☐	☐	☐
6 Explains method and timing of depot injections:			
Initial need for test dose	☐	☐	☐
Injections initially given with slow reduction of tablets	☐	☐	☐
Injection made up of 2 to 3 ml oily solution	☐	☐	☐
Injection sites rotated to avoid local complications	☐	☐	☐
Need to titrate dose to suit the individual, which may take several months	☐	☐	☐

*Once suitable dose is found injections
are given every 2–4 weeks* ☐ ☐ ☐

7 Explains local and systemic side-effects ☐ ☐ ☐

8 Gives clear, jargon-free explanation ☐ ☐ ☐

9 Checks patient's understanding of
information ☐ ☐ ☐

10 Systematic and organised ☐ ☐ ☐

SP to mark

11 This doctor was supportive ☐ ☐ ☐

STATION 2.42

The major antipsychotic and antidepressive medications have numerous side-effects which often overlap. The most appropriate drug combination and dosage must be tailored for the individual.

1 (E) (g)

Lithium has a narrow therapeutic range and its plasma levels should be closely monitored. The normal lithium therapeutic range to aim for is between 0.4 to 1 mmol^{-1}. Toxicity occurs at levels of 1.5 mmol^{-1} and severe, life-threatening toxicity occurs at 2 mmol^{-1}. Lithium has many side-effects and the decision to use it should be taken by an expert with plasma-monitoring facilities available. All patients on lithium should be issued with a lithium card

Regular side-effects of lithium (1.5–2.0 mmol^{-1})

Early changes are non-specific and include agitation and apathy which may be confused with signs of worsening of the underlying condition.

- Nephrogenic diabetes insipidus (polyuria/polydypsia)
- Neurological: fine tremor (may become coarse), decreasing level of consciousness, confusion, dysarthria, dizziness
- Gastrointestinal disturbances: vomiting, diarrhoea, anorexia, weight gain and oedema

Severe side-effects of lithium (> 2 mmol^{-1})

- Neurological: hyperextension of limbs, hyper-reflexia, seizures
- Psychiatric: confusion, toxic psychoses
- Circulatory collapse: shock
- Hypothyroidism ± goitre
- Raised ADH
- Hypokalaemia with associated ECG changes
- Renal failure

Toxicity should be treated by withdrawal of the drug and, if renal impairment is associated, haemodialysis should be considered. Hypovolaemia, circulatory collapse and electrolyte imbalance should be corrected. Diabetes insipidus and hypothyroidism should be treated in the usual ways.

2 **(F) (c)**

SSRIs such as fluoxetine, paroxetine, sertraline and citalopram are antidepressants. They have less sedative effect and are less cardiotoxic than the tricyclic antidepressants and are therefore particularly useful in the elderly. The mechanism of hyponatraemia is unclear but is thought to be due to SIADH. It is one of the commonest reasons to stop their use in elderly patients who often have concurrent diuretic therapy which also causes hyponatraemia.

3 **(A) (d)**

Amitriptyline is a tricyclic antidepressant used in depressive conditions particularly where sedation is required. It has several side-effects including anticholinergic, cardiovascular, haematological and psychiatric effects. It may cause agranulocytosis, thrombocytopenia and eosinophilia, as well as hyponatraemia and derangement of the LFTs.

4 **(B) (f)**

The neuroleptic malignant syndrome may arise with phenothiazines (eg chlorpromazine), butyrophenones (eg haloperidol) and rarely with tricyclic antidepressants. It is characterised by a high fever, fluctuating level of consciousness, muscle rigidity and autonomic dysfunction such as urinary incontinence and resting tachycardia. The diagnosis should be suspected from the history and confirmed by grossly elevated CK levels and negative sepsis screen (the principal differential). Treatment should include withdrawal of the drug and supportive measures, including nutrition, intravenous fluids and urinary catheterisation.

5 **(G) (b)**

The phenothiazines are principally used in the treatment of schizophrenia and other psychoses. They have multiple side-effects including extrapyramidal movement disorders, for which procyclidine is given, anticholinergic effects, cardiovascular, endocrine and haematological effects. They may also cause derangement of the LFTs and cholestatic jaundice.

Answers

6 **(C) (e)**

Phenelzine is a MAOI. Their use is restricted because of the interactions they have with food substances such as cheese and yeast extracts, alcoholic drinks, and other drugs, particularly indirect-acting sympathomimetics such as nasal decongestants and cough mixtures. They should not be given with the other classes of antidepressants as this too may lead to sympathomimetic effects. These interactions may precipitate dangerous rises in blood pressure, usually signalled by a severe, throbbing headache. All patients on MAOIs should be issued with a warning card explaining these interactions.

A less common side-effect is peripheral neuropathy, similar to that caused by isoniazid.

7 **(D) (a)**

Flupenthixol is principally used in depot injections for the long-term control of schizophrenia. As with chlorpromazine it has multiple side-effects and may cause endocrine effects including hyperprolactinaemia, galactorrhoea and menstrual irregularity.

Chapter 3:
Ophthalmology and
Otolaryngology Answers

Chapter 3

Ophthalmology and Otolaryngology Answers

STATION 3.1

Patient history

I woke up on Monday morning (four days ago) with a very itchy right eye. I kept rubbing it and the next day my left eye was red and felt gritty and was watering. I tried washing my eyes under the tap but it didn't help much.

Two boys from my scout troop also had red eyes when we returned from a weekend 'outward bound' trip. We had spent two days camping in the forest and swam in the stream. My mother thinks I may have picked up a bug in camp.

I had a squint when I was young and had to wear glasses with a black patch on one side for a long time. My eyes are alright now.

Assessment	Good	Adequate	Poor/not done
1 Appropriate introduction (full name and role)	☐	☐	☐
2 Establishes severity and duration of symptoms	☐	☐	☐
3 Checks symptom progression and/or complications	☐	☐	☐
4 Enquires into causative or associated factors	☐	☐	☐
5 Asks about relieving factors or remedial measures	☐	☐	☐
6 Establishes past medical history	☐	☐	☐
7 Makes reasonable attempt at a working diagnosis	☐	☐	☐
8 Uses an appropriate questioning type	☐	☐	☐
9 Summarises history back to the patient	☐	☐	☐
10 Systematic and organised approach	☐	☐	☐

Comment

Four main causes of painful, red eyes are:

- Conjunctivitis
- Blepharitis (inflammation of lid margins with secondary ocular irritation)
- Allergic reactions
- Dysthyroid eye disease

The relevant questions are:

- Is there a discharge? Mucopurulent discharge is associated with bacterial conjunctivitis
- Is the patient atopic? He may be prone to allergic reactions in response to pollen, house dust or animal hair
- Is the patient hyperthyroid?

In conjunctivitis, the conjunctiva is usually diffusely red and haemorrhages may be present. The inflammation usually starts in one eye before infecting the other. The discharge may be purulent in bacterial infection and watery in viral infection or in atopic allergies. Pain is unusual while discomfort and irritation are common.

STATION 3.2

1 (D) (e) (H)
Keratoconjunctivitis sicca is part of the 'dry' sicca syndrome associated with lacrimal and salivary gland infiltration by lymphocytes. The dry eye should be protected with hypromellose eye drops, which act as artificial tears, lubricating the cornea.

2 (E) (d) (J)
Anterior uveitis or iritis is associated with several systemic disorders including ankylosing spondylitis, Reiter's syndrome, Behçet's disease and sarcoidosis. It may be associated with pupillary constriction.

3 (A) (c) (G)
Bacterial conjunctivitis is commonly caused by *Staphylococcus aureus*, *Haemophilus influenzae* and *Streptococcus pneumoniae*. Less common infections include gonococcus, trachoma, toxoplasmosis, and adeno and herpes viruses.

4 (B) (a) (I)
Scleritis and episcleritis are associated with rheumatoid arthritis and Wegener's granulomatosis. It may lead to scleromalacia and perforation if left untreated.

5 (C) (b) (F)
HSV-1 and HSV-2 may both cause eye infection, although HSV-1 is predominantly responsible. The infection should be treated with topical acyclovir or vidarabine.

Comment
Acute glaucoma is one of the most serious and sinister causes of red eye. The eye is often very painful and feels hard and uncomfortable. If glaucoma is suspected, an urgent ophthalmological opinion should be sought.

Answers

STATION 3.3

Patient history

I grind and polish gem stones and work on an electric lathe. My left eye became sore a couple of days ago and the pain is getting worse. My sight in that eye has become blurred and I find that the glare hurts the eye. I wear a magnifying eye-piece on my right eye when at work. My eyesight has been excellent and I do not wear spectacles. My general health is good except for a long-standing stomach ulcer for which I am on ranitidine. There is a history of glaucoma in the family. My mother and an older sister have this condition.

I am worried about whether I am getting the same condition and about what it means for my work. I am dependent on having good eyesight.

Assessment	Good	Adequate	Poor/not done
1 Appropriate introduction (full name and role)	☐	☐	☐
2 Explains purpose of the interview	☐	☐	☐
3 Establishes severity and duration of symptoms	☐	☐	☐
4 Establishes symptom progression and/or complications	☐	☐	☐
5 Enquires into causative/associated factors	☐	☐	☐
6 Asks about relieving factors or remedial measures.	☐	☐	☐
7 Establishes past medical history	☐	☐	☐
8 Elicits patient's concerns and responds sensitively	☐	☐	☐
9 Uses an appropriate questioning technique	☐	☐	☐
10 Summarises history back to the patient, including concerns	☐	☐	☐
11 Systematic and organised approach	☐	☐	☐
12 Makes a reasonable attempt at a working diagnosis	☐	☐	☐

Answers

Comment

Questions to ask are:

1 Was the patient involved in activity associated with a high risk of corneal foreign body?
2 Is there a history of trauma to the eye?
3 Is looking at bright light painful?
4 Is vision blurred? (This is common in the painful red eye due to excess watering or a central corneal abrasion. Acute glaucoma causes corneal clouding and is a frequent cause in the elderly.)
5 Does the patient wear contact lenses? (Overworn or poorly cleaned contact lenses may induce corneal abrasion or ulcers.)
6 Has the patient had iritis (eye inflammation) in the past?
7 Has the patient had an eye operation recently? (Irritation to corneal sutures following cataract or squint surgery may produce a red, painful eye.)

STATION 3.4

1   fig 3.4a   Hyphaema
    fig 3.4b   Iridocyclitis
    fig 3.4c   Retinal oedema and haemorrhage
    fig 3.4d   Papilloedema

2   Traumatic iritis
    Glaucoma
    Dislocated lens or cataract
    Vitreous haemorrhage
    Retinal tear leading to retinal detachment
    Choroidal rupture
    Scleral rupture
    Optic nerve injury

3   **True**: (a), (c), (d)
    False: (b), (c)

Comment

Blunt injury to the eyeball causes compression of the iris by aqueous humour, causing a hyphaema or pressure increase in the posterior chamber, producing vitreous haemorrhage, retinal tear or scleral rupture. A 'blow out' fracture is when the compression force also causes the orbital floor to fracture. Initial treatment is to apply eye patches to both eyes to decrease eye movement, and the administration of diuretics and/or steroids to decrease intraocular pressure

STATION 3.5

fig 3.5a   Convergent squint (left eye). Refractory correction
fig 3.5b   Acute conjunctivitis
                  Wash the eyes with normal saline or tap water
fig 3.5c   Dysthyroid eye disease
                  Exposure keratitis (diplopia, cranial nerve palsies III, IV VI,
                  secondary glaucoma)
fig 3.5d   Retinoblastoma
                  Pupillary white reflex

Comment

Retinoblastoma is usually detected during the first year of life. The patient is brought
to the clinic on account of the peculiar white or yellow reflex 'amaurotic cat's eye'.
The tumour is multicentric, affecting the other eye in a quarter of the patients.
Extension along the optic nerve to the brain is common. Treatment is removal of the
eye with a long length of the optic nerve. Exenteration of the orbit is required in
locally advanced tumours. The prognosis is usually dismal.

STATION 3.6

1 Grave's orbitopathy
2 Exophthalmos or dysthyroid eye disease
3 Double vision
   Exposure keratitis
   Retinal or optic neuronal vascular impairment and secondary glaucoma
4 High doses of steroids with/without immunosuppressive agents
   Ensure lid closure at night by lid taping
   May require tarsorrhaphy or orbital decompression

Comment

Exophthalmos in Grave's disease is caused by exophthalmos-producing factor
secreted by the hypothalamus. The condition does not always regress with control of
the hyperthyroid state. When ophthalmoplegia or chemosis threatens vision, orbital
decompression may be required. Systemic corticosteroids are often beneficial in
reducing orbital oedema. In severe cases local radiotherapy to the orbit is required.

STATION 3.7

1 Chalazion (meibomian or tarsal cyst)
2 (A) Chalazion clamp   (C) Curette
   (B) Scalpel   (D) Fine scissors
3 Equipment layout: chalazion clamp, chalazion curette, fine scissors and forceps,
   scalpel (No 11 and 15 blades), anaesthetic eye drops (amethocaine 1% of
   oxynuprocaine 0.4%), local anaesthetic for injection (0.5% Marcain or 1%
   lidocaine), antibiotic eye ointment, eyepad

   - Anaesthetise conjunctiva with drops
   - local infiltration of anaesthetic agent (1–2ml) around swelling
   - Apply clamp so that cyst protrudes on conjunctival surface
   - Vertical conjunctival incision into cyst
   - Curette contents
   - Instil antibiotic ointment
   - Apply eyepad over closed eye and apply pressure for 10 minutes
   - Postoperative care: bathe eye daily and instil ointment twice daily for three
     days

Comment

Inflammation of the glands of the eyelid results in a chalazion (meibomian cyst).
They present as an acute or chronic swelling of the lid; spontaneous resolution is
rare. Treatment is surgical; the conjunctival sac is well anaesthetised along with the
lid. The latter is everted and a vertical incision is made at the point of greatest
discolouration. The cavity is evacuated and curetted. The procedure is repeated if
granulation tissue develops in the wound. A stye is an infection of an eyelash follicle.

STATION 3.8

1 Cataract
2 Congenital: infantile, Down's syndrome, dystrophic myotonia
   Metabolic: diabetes, galactosaemia, hypocalcaemia
   Steroid induced
   Physical causes (eg injury)
   Secondary to other eye disease
   Skin diseases: atopic dermatitis
   Senility
3 Maturity of a cataract
4 Surgical extraction of cataract, with intraocular lens implant

Comment

No medical measures are useful in the treatment of cataract once lens opacities have developed. In acquired cataract a metabolic cause such as diabetes mellitus must be looked for and treated. Surgical removal is indicated when the cataract is mature. In the meantime, the refraction should be corrected at frequent intervals as it deteriorates. Advice should be given on adequate illumination for reading.

A secondary cataract is when the opacity returns following lens extraction. This is due to part of the lens cortex sticking to the capsule and subsequently proliferating, especially when the cataract is not mature. Further surgery is usually indicated.

STATION 3.9

Assessment	Good	Adequate	Poor/not done
1 Appropriate introduction (full name and role)	☐	☐	☐
2 Obtains verbal consent and explains context of visual examination	☐	☐	☐
3 Visual acuity: ensures patient is seated 6 m from the chart	☐	☐	☐
4 Asks patient to close one eye and read the chart line by line	☐	☐	☐
5 Repeats the procedure for the other eye	☐	☐	☐
6 Visual field test: instructs the patient to look at the examiner's face covering the other eye	☐	☐	☐
7 Examiner introduces a moving object (a hand) from the periphery from different angles and asks the patient to indicate when it comes into vision (see fig 3.9)	☐	☐	☐
8 Repeats the procedure on the other eye	☐	☐	☐
9 Completes examination and thanks patient	☐	☐	☐
10 Presents findings in a clear, sequential manner	☐	☐	☐

Answers

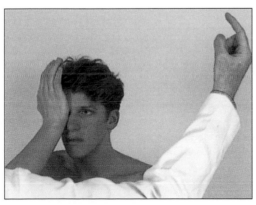

fig 3.9

Comment

Examination of the central vision is tested by using the letter sets on a Snellen chart at a distance of six metres. Vision is expressed as a fraction of the normal – the latter being 6/6, if the patient only sees the letter twice its size, visual acuity is 6/12. (These figures are written on each line of the chart.)

The visual fields can be quickly assessed by the confrontation test, in which the patient closes one eye, looking straight with the other eye into the corresponding eye of the doctor. The doctor's moving finger is introduced in turn from the periphery in the four diagonal positions, and the patient indicates once the movement is seen. A more precise test is carried out by perimetry, where the visual fields are mapped.

Assessment of visual acuity is fundamental in any eye disorder as it measures visual function.

Visual fields testing indicates the site of a lesion. Testing using finger movements peripherally shows severe defects. The detection of red colour is more sensitive as this tends to be affected earlier (a red object may be used).

STATION 3.10

1 (D) (g)
Wilson's disease is due to an abnormality of copper metabolism, centred in the biliary tree, leading to ectopic deposition within the viscera. The common sites include the liver, eye, basal ganglia, myocardium and kidneys.

The Kayser–Fleischer rings are pathognomonic and appear as grey corneal rings in dark eyes and brown rings in light-coloured eyes.

2 (H) (e)
Down's syndrome (trisomy 21) is associated with several eye abnormalities, including epicanthic folds, keratoconus, brushfield spots and infantile cataracts.

3 (A) (f)
Marfan's syndrome is an autosomal dominant disorder due to abnormalities within the fibrillin gene on chromosome 15. Fibrillin is an important component of several connective tissues, including the suspensory ligament of the lens. The abnormality classically causes superior dislocation of the lens, unlike homocystinuria, a similar clinical condition, which causes downward dislocation. The unsupported iris wobbles with movement, termed 'iridodonesis'.

4 (G) (a)

Pingueculae are subconjunctival areas of yellowish brown. These are raised, yellowish-white areas that occur, usually nasally around the limbus of the eye. They are often bilateral and predominantly occur in middle to old age. They are usually benign but may be associated with Gaucher's disease, in which they may have a more brown pigmentation.

5 (B) (d)

Tuberous sclerosis is an autosomal dominant disorder but commonly arises through spontaneous mutation. It is associated with the classical triad of adenoma sebaceum, epilepsy and severe mental retardation. Retinal phacomas are glial masses seen on retinoscopy. Other common lesions include shagreen patches and ash leaf spots.

6 (C) (b)

Angioid streaks are irregular grey lines radiating out from the optic disc. They may occur in pseudoxanthoma elasticum, Paget's disease of the bone, sickle cell disease and Ehlers–Danlos syndrome. They may be associated with blue sclera in pseudoxanthoma.

7 (F) (h)

Cherry red spots occur in several of the sphingolipidoses, including Neimann–Pick and Tay–Sachs disease. They arise due to the abnormal sphingolipid accumulation within the ganglion cells centred within the macula.

8 (E) (c)

Blue or pigmented sclera arise in several disorders, including osteogenesis imperfecta, pseudoxanthoma elasticum and alkaptonuria. This list, and the answers to the 'red eye' in Station 3.2 emphasise the importance of the clinical examination of the eye. For diagnosing common conditions, such as anaemia and jaundice, to hereditary disorders, the eye should not be overlooked.

Answers

STATION 3.11

Patient history

I am 65 years old and a retired car salesman. I had a heart attack 12 years ago and have long-standing diabetes mellitus, which is controlled with diet and tablets. I also have high blood pressure.

In the last six months I have had four or five episodes of dizziness associated with vomiting. The last episode was two weeks ago. I attended the Emergency Department and they referred me to this clinic.

The episodes come on suddenly with no obvious cause. The last one started while I was just sitting and reading the newspaper. It's as if the whole world is spinning round, like being drunk. It doesn't get any better if I stand up or lie down, or if I move my head, although this makes me feel more nauseated. I have been sick a few times. I have no other neurological symptoms and haven't had any tinnitus or deafness. The episodes last five to six hours and then just go away.

I am taking atenolol for my blood pressure and heart problem. I stopped taking aspirin tablets about a year ago because I felt I did not need them any more. I am worried by this. I have been looking forward to retirement and wondering whether I'm now seriously ill.

Assessment	Good	Adequate	Poor/not done
1 Appropriate introduction (full name and role)	☐	☐	☐
2 Explains what interview is to be about and asks for consent	☐	☐	☐
3 Establishes duration of presenting complaint	☐	☐	☐
4 Establishes what the patient means by dizziness (ie vertigo)	☐	☐	☐
5 Establishes/excludes the characteristics of vertigo:			
Onset – acute or insidious	☐	☐	☐

Pattern – continuous or episodic	☐	☐	☐
Duration of episodes	☐	☐	☐
Relieving factors	☐	☐	☐
Exacerbating factors	☐	☐	☐
Associated auditory problems (ie deafness, tinnitus)	☐	☐	☐
Other neurological symptoms (ie diplopia, dysarthria, ataxia)	☐	☐	☐
Associated nausea and vomiting	☐	☐	☐
6 Establishes previous medical history, ie hypertension, CVA, IHD, DM	☐	☐	☐
7 Establishes treatment history (ie excludes drugs causing postural hypotension)	☐	☐	☐
8 Establishes patient's concerns and responds sensitively	☐	☐	☐
9 Uses an appropriate questioning technique	☐	☐	☐
10 Avoids or explains jargon	☐	☐	☐
11 Summarises history back to the patient	☐	☐	☐
12 Systematic, organised approach	☐	☐	☐
13 Makes a reasonable attempt at a diagnosis	☐	☐	☐

Diagnosis

Vertebrobasilar transient ischaemic attacks.

Answers

STATION 3.12

Patient history

I am married and work as a medical secretary at a private clinic in town. I woke up this morning bleeding from the nose with blood all over the pillow and the bed-sheet. I could not stop the bleeding with finger pressure over the bridge of the nose. I have had nose bleeds in childhood and early teens but had grown out of it. At the time my doctors could not find a cause for it.

I have always been in excellent health except during my two pregnancies four and six years ago when I developed pre-eclampsia and was put on tablets to control my blood pressure. I stopped taking these two to three months after the birth of my children. When I was pregnant I had kidney and bladder infections which cleared on antibiotics. I am presently not on any medications.

Assessment	Good	Adequate	Poor/not done
1 Appropriate introduction (full name and role)	☐	☐	☐
2 Explains the purpose of the interview and asks for consent	☐	☐	☐
3 Establishes severity and duration of symptoms	☐	☐	☐
4 Establishes symptom progression and/or complications	☐	☐	☐
5 Enquires into causative/associated factors	☐	☐	☐
6 Asks about relieving factors or remedial measures	☐	☐	☐
7 Establishes past medical history	☐	☐	☐
8 Makes a reasonable attempt at a working diagnosis	☐	☐	☐
9 Uses an appropriate questioning technique	☐	☐	☐
10 Summarises history back to the patient	☐	☐	☐
11 Systematic organised approach	☐	☐	☐

Comment

Nose bleeds may be due to local or systemic causes. Patients who are hypertensive do not bleed more often but when epistaxis occurs it may be more severe and may require admission. Bleeding uncontrolled by external pressure requires gauze packing or balloon compression for 24–48 h with bed rest and sedation.

In the young patient bleeding is usually from the anterior aspect of the nasal septum (Little's area) and the bleeding area moves posteriorly with age. Other systemic causes are familial telangiectasia (Osler's disease), blood dyscrasias and anticoagulant therapy.

Answers

STATION 3.13

History from parent

We are staying at a holiday camp and Susie became listless three days ago and then started running a fever, developed a sore throat and has become hoarse and is losing her voice. I have been giving her two teaspoonfuls of Calpol every few hours but last night she became hot, flushed and breathless and I am very worried that she is now catching her breath and coughing hurts her throat. I think she is quite ill and this is frightening.

Susie has had chest infections in the past when she had the 'flu but she has never had problems with her breathing. She has always been an active child and her health has been very good on the whole. She was a premature baby and was nursed in an incubator for nearly a month when she was born.

Assessment	Good	Adequate	Poor/not done
1 Appropriate introduction (full name and role)	☐	☐	☐
2 Explains what interview will be about	☐	☐	☐
3 Establishes severity and duration of symptoms	☐	☐	☐
4 Establishes symptom progression and/or complications	☐	☐	☐
5 Enquires into causative/associated factors	☐	☐	☐
6 Asks about relieving factors or remedial measures	☐	☐	☐
7 Establishes past medical history	☐	☐	☐
8 Elicits mother's concerns and responds sensitively	☐	☐	☐
9 Uses an appropriate questioning technique	☐	☐	☐
10 Summarises history back to the mother	☐	☐	☐
11 Involves the child and mother in the interview	☐	☐	☐

12 Systematic and organised approach ☐ ☐ ☐

13 Makes a reasonable attempt at a working
    diagnosis ☐ ☐ ☐

Comment

Acute tonsillitis is a pyogenic infection of the tonsillar lymph nodes caused usually by group A haemolytic *Streptococcus spp*. It is characterised by sore throat, hoarseness, dysphagia and fever. There may be cervical lymphadenopathy (jugulo-digastric nodes). White pustules may be visible on the surface of the palatine tonsils.

Recurrent infection, particularly if this is over an 18–24 month period, is an indication for tonsillectomy.

Surgery is also indicated for airway obstruction, peritonsillar abscess and the sleep apnoea syndrome. There is no evidence of long-term immunological sequelae following tonsillectomy.

STATION 3.14

(A) 1 Right-sided LMN facial nerve palsy
     2 Ask the patient to whistle, smile and frown or grimace
     Attempt to open the eyelids against resistance

(B) All are **True**

Comment

In upper motor neurone lesions of the facial nerve, the lower part of the face is more severely affected. Recovery is usual and precedes that of the limbs on the affected side. In lower motor neurone lesions the weakness is to the same extent in both the upper and lower halves of the face. Paralysis is often severe, causing facial asymmetry at rest. Tears and saliva may drip down that side. Bell's palsy is unilateral and is of sudden onset and presumed to be an immune response, producing facial nerve swelling and resultant compression in the narrow confines of the temporal bone. Complete or partial recovery is usual. Steroid therapy is indicated within the first 48 h of onset.

STATION 3.15

1 Pleomorphic adenoma of the parotid gland, mixed cellular histological pattern
2 Conservative, superficial parotidectomy
3 Facial palsy; identify and preserve the facial nerve trunk and its branches during surgery
4 Carcinoma of the parotid gland

Comment

A swelling of the parotid gland must be distinguished from other swellings in the cheek and anterior triangle of the neck, the most common being enlarged lymph nodes. Pleomorphic adenomas are benign but may become malignant after a period of many years. Fine needle aspiration cytology of the lesion is to be avoided, due to the risk of tumour implantation in the subcutaneous tissue. Enucleation of the tumour from its false capsule results in recurrence, and treatment is by parotidectomy; the facial nerve and its branches that are present within the gland must be identified and preserved. Most parotid tumours lie superficial to the facial nerve branches and a superficial conservative parotidectomy is performed. When the deep part of the gland is involved, great care must be taken to preserve the overlying nerves when resecting the tumour.

STATION 3.16

History from foster mother

Timmy has been irritable for the past four days and has been off his food. He was running a fever yesterday and was violently sick this morning. He keeps holding his left ear and crying. He wouldn't let me get near his ear and he goes into tantrums. I am at my wits' end coping with him and he refuses to take his Calpol syrup. I have had him for a little over a year and he has had the odd cold and 'flu and tummy upset. His mother told me that he was a well baby and has had all his vaccinations. She didn't say anything about having ear problems.

Assessment	Good	Adequate	Poor/not done
1 Appropriate introduction (full name and role)	☐	☐	☐
2 Establishes severity and duration of symptoms	☐	☐	☐
3 Establishes symptom progression and/or complications	☐	☐	☐
4 Enquires into causative/associated factors	☐	☐	☐
5 Asks about relieving factors or remedial measures	☐	☐	☐
6 Establishes past medical history	☐	☐	☐
7 Uses an appropriate questioning technique	☐	☐	☐
8 Summarises history back to the foster mother	☐	☐	☐
9 Involves the child in the interview	☐	☐	☐
10 Systematic and organised approach	☐	☐	☐
11 Makes a reasonable attempt at a working diagnosis	☐	☐	☐

Comment

Acute suppurative otitis media (middle ear infection) in children usually follows a recurrent upper respiratory tract infection. Initially there is an inflammation of the eustachian tube progressing to inflammation of the tympanic membrane. Otoscopy reveals a red, lustreless bulging drum. Untreated, the infection may lead to perforation of the drum or spread to the air cells in the mastoid or petrous temporal bone.

A persisting and discharge indicates chronicity (glue ear) and may present with hearing loss, recurrent ear infections, developmental or behavioural problems.

STATION 3.17

Assessment	Good	Adequate	Poor/not done
1 Appropriate introduction (full name and role)	☐	☐	☐
2 Explains examination and obtains verbal consent	☐	☐	☐
3 Ensures patient is seated and requests to hold head still during examination	☐	☐	☐
4 Inspects pinna and external meatus	☐	☐	☐
5 Introduces otoscope with gentle traction on pinna	☐	☐	☐
6 Ensures comfort on completion and thanks patient	☐	☐	☐
7 Presents findings in a logical and sequential manner	☐	☐	☐

Comment

The positioning of the auroscope and technique of examination are important as injury to the external meatus and the drum may be caused by injudicious movement (fig 3.17). Children may require sedation.

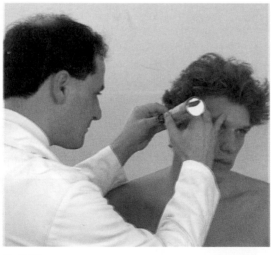

fig 3.17

STATION 3.18

Assessment	Good	Adequate	Poor/not done
1 Appriopriate introduction (full name and role)	☐	☐	☐
2 Explains examination to patient. Gains verbal consent	☐	☐	☐
3 Candidate washes their hands using the alcohol handwash provided (no marks if candidate only expresses the need to wash if handwash is provided)	☐	☐	☐
4 Exposes the whole of the neck including the full length of both clavicles. Positions the patient so they can be examined from the front and behind	☐	☐	☐
5 If not obvious asks the patient where the lump is and whether it is tender, how long it's been there and whether it changes in size	☐	☐	☐
6 Conducts examination from behind			
Describes submental, submandibular, parotid, postauricular and occipital nodes or absence, and palpates along the external jugular vein from the angle of the mandible to middle of the clavicle then along the internal jugular vein particularly in the jugular diagastric region and mid-cervical region where the internal jugular vein is crossed by the omohyoid muscle	☐	☐	☐
7 Examines behind the medial and middle thirds of the clavicle picking up the lax lower end of the sternomastoid muscle to identify a lymph node situated deep to this structure	☐	☐	☐
8 Examines along anterior surface of the neck for anterior jugular and prelaryngeal lymph nodes	☐	☐	☐

Answers

9 Once lump is identified describes site,
   size, shape and surface, colour,
   temperature, tenderness, mobility ☐   ☐   ☐

10 Describes interior consistency:
   compressibility, reducibility, cough,
   impulse, fluid, thrill, indentation,
   fluctuation, discharge, pulsation,
   expansion, transillumination, bruit ☐   ☐   ☐

11 Describes surroundings: induration,
   tethering, invasion of the nerves, vessels,
   other tissues, nodes and related diseases ☐   ☐   ☐

12 Repositions patient to ensure dignity,
   covers and comforts, and thanks them ☐   ☐   ☐

13 Presents findings in a fluent logical
   manner ☐   ☐   ☐

14 Gives a differential diagnosis and
   possible causes ☐   ☐   ☐

Chapter 4:
Urology and Renal
Medicine Answers

Chapter 4

Urology and Renal Medicine Answers

STATION 4.1

Patient history

I am 18 years old and, for the last five years, I have been getting recurrent urinary symptoms. I have had multiple urinary infections, blood in my urine and, more recently, dull pain in my lower back. In the last 18 months I have also had recurrent headaches and visual disturbance. My mother and grandmother both had kidney disease and my mother died of a bleed inside the brain. Each episode of infection is relieved for a week or two by antibiotics but I have had to self-medicate from time to time to stop them coming back so frequently. Each infection lasts for 5–6 days with frequency, as well as pain and blood when I pass urine. I have been admitted on three occasions with severe infections with associated fever and rigors.

I have never been further investigated because I am terrified of the possible diagnoses and have always taken my own discharge before the hospital has had time to do any secondary investigations. I have also moved around a lot because of my father's job in the Navy. I have not met this GP before.

Assessment	Good	Adequate	Poor/not done
1 Appropriate introduction (full name and role)	☐	☐	☐
2 Establishes reason for patient's visit	☐	☐	☐
3 Establishes duration of urinary problems	☐	☐	☐
4 Establishes symptoms of urinary tract infection	☐	☐	☐
5 Establishes associated fever and rigors	☐	☐	☐

6 Establishes symptoms of polycystic
kidney disease :

   Loin pain □ □

   Haematuria □ □

   Features of hypertension □ □

7 Establishes family history of renal disease □ □

8 Establishes mother died of subarachnoid
haemorrhage □ □ □

9 Elicits patient's concerns and responds
sensitively □ □ □

10 Uses an appropriate questioning
technique □ □ □

11 Avoids or explains jargon □ □ □

12 Summarises history back to the patient,
including concerns □ □ □

13 Systematic, organised approach □ □ □

14 Makes reasonable attempt at a diagnosis □ □ □

SP to mark

15 The doctor was empathic □ □ □

Diagnosis

Recurrent urinary tract infection presenting secondary to probable adult polycystic
kidney disease.

STATION 4.2

Patient history

I am 24 years old and am normally fit and well. I have come to the Emergency Department with severe left-sided pain in my lower back. I have had the pain now for eight hours and it has gradually increased in intensity and is now unbearable. The pain comes and goes in waves and has no radiation. I have had two similar episodes in the last year, but these were not as severe. I have not had any symptoms of urinary infection, fever, or rigors or pain on passing urine.

Assessment	Good	Adequate	Poor/not done
1 Appropriate introduction (full name and role)	☐	☐	☐
2 Explains purpose of interview	☐	☐	☐
3 Establishes duration of present illness	☐	☐	☐
4 Establishes left-sided loin pain	☐	☐	☐
5 Establishes character and nature of the pain	☐	☐	☐
6 Establishes history of two similar but less severe episodes	☐	☐	☐
7 Excludes symptoms of UTI	☐	☐	☐
8 Asks about passage of renal stones	☐	☐	☐
9 Uses an appropriate questioning technique	☐	☐	☐
10 Avoids or explains jargon	☐	☐	☐
11 Summarises history back to patient	☐	☐	☐
11 Makes a reasonable attempt at a diagnosis	☐	☐	☐
12 Talks competently about the management options	☐	☐	☐

Answers

Diagnosis

Renal colic secondary to renal stones.

Comment

Renal stones produce intense, acute pain, causing the patient to roll around in agony. The most important acute treatments are adequate analgesia, with either pethidine or voltarol, and IV fluids. When using pethidine, or if vomiting is present, an anti-emetic should also be given. Initial management should include FBC, U+Es, LFTs, amylase and calcium, plain AXR, IV access and IV fluids. An IVU should be organised as soon as is possible.

Small stones may pass spontaneously and the patient may have noticed previous stones passed in the urine. Larger stones may require surgical removal or may be disintegrated using lithotripsy.

STATION 4.3

Patient history

I am the wife of the patient, who is 55 years old and a diabetic. He has non-insulin dependent diabetes mellitus and hypertension, and was recently started on an ACE inhibitor by his local GP on the advice of the hospital.

In the last week he has become increasingly confused and unwell. He has been vomiting and has had severe hiccups. He is continually scratching and I have not seen him pass any urine for over 48 h. His ankles are becoming increasingly swollen. He does not have any other systemic symptoms. He is known to have slight kidney problems due to diabetes and his high blood pressure. As well as the ACE inhibitor he is on gliclazide and bendrofluazide. I am upset that he is feeling so ill, and worried that he won't pull through this.

Assessment	Good	Adequate	Poor/not done
1 Appropriate introduction (full name and role)	☐	☐	☐
2 Explains purpose of interview and checks relationship with patient	☐	☐	☐
3 Establishes the premorbid problems of the patient	☐	☐	☐
4 Establishes medications and recent addition of ACE inhibitor therapy	☐	☐	☐
5 Establishes duration of present illness	☐	☐	☐
6 Establishes/excludes symptoms of uraemia and renal failure:			
Nausea and vomiting		☐	☐
Pruritis		☐	☐
Hiccups		☐	☐
Oliguria in the last week		☐	☐
Peripheral oedema		☐	☐
7 Elicits patient's concerns and responds sensitively	☐	☐	☐

8 Uses an appropriate questioning technique	☐	☐	☐
9 Avoids or explains jargon	☐	☐	☐
10 Summarises history back to the patient, including concerns	☐	☐	☐
11 Makes a reasonable attempt at a diagnosis	☐	☐	☐
12 Discusses the management in a competent manner	☐	☐	☐
13 Systematic, organised approach	☐	☐	☐

Diagnosis

Uraemic precoma, secondary to acute on chronic renal failure. The recent addition of the ACE inhibitor has precipitated the dramatic acceleration of his renal impairment.

Answers

STATION 4.4

Patient history

I am a 53-year-old bank manager and have been fit and well until five months ago. Initially I noticed occasional episodes of blood mixed with my urine but, more recently, I have had several episodes of passing blood. This is associated with a dull pain in my left loin and I have also noticed a slight swelling in this area. I have lost several kilogrammes in weight and have a poor appetite. I have had no energy to do anything and feel continually tired. In the last few weeks I have also had a fever particularly at night, and have woken on several occasions drenched in sweat. I am worried that something is seriously wrong. My work is now being affected and I have a lot of responsibilities.

Assessment	Good	Adequate	Poor/not done
1 Appropriate introduction (full name and role)	☐	☐	☐
2 Explains purpose of the interview	☐	☐	☐
3 Establishes the duration of the presenting illness	☐	☐	☐
4 Establishes the nature of the haematuria, ie frank blood	☐	☐	☐
5 Establishes frequency of the haematuria	☐	☐	☐
6 Establishes associated dull left loin pain and swelling	☐	☐	☐
7 Establishes associated malaise, lethargy, anorexia and weight loss	☐	☐	☐
8 Establishes history of night sweats	☐	☐	☐
9 Elicits patient's concerns and responds sensitively	☐	☐	☐
10 Uses an appropriate questioning technique	☐	☐	☐
11 Avoids or explains jargon	☐	☐	☐
12 Summarises history back to the patient, including concerns	☐	☐	☐

13 Makes a reasonable attempt at a diagnosis	☐	☐	☐
14 Is able to discuss the possible further management in a clear and competent manner	☐	☐	☐
15 Systematic, organised approach	☐	☐	☐

Diagnosis

Malignant renal tumour.

Comment

Any patient over 40 years old with painless haematuria must have malignancy of the renal tract excluded. Blood tests should include a FBC to exclude anaemia secondary to haematuria or polcythaemia, which is a rarer presentation. U+Es may be abnormal, particularly in bilateral disease. The ESR is often raised. A CXR, USS of the renal tract and an IVU should be routinely performed to assess the tumour and its spread.

Renal tumours are often extremely vascular and may be demonstrated using renal arteriography. A staging CT scan of the abdomen should also be performed in this situation.

Unilateral tumours are generally treated by surgical excision. Radiotherapy and chemotherapy are also used, particularly in bilateral and metastatic disease.

Answers

STATION 4.5

Patient history

I am 37 years old and have had SLE for the last six years. I have recently noticed my ankles and calves swelling up, to such an extent in the last few weeks that I now cannot get my shoes on. In the last ten days I have not passed very much urine, despite drinking a lot of fluids and have also become breathless on exertion. Other than the SLE I have had no serious illnesses and have never had any problems with my heart. At present I am taking azathioprine and steroids for the SLE. I am worried that my SLE is getting worse and that I'm not going to be able to care properly for my children.

Assessment	Good	Adequate	Poor/not done
1 Appropriate introduction (full name and role)	☐	☐	☐
2 Explains purpose of the interview	☐	☐	☐
3 Establishes the presenting problem	☐	☐	☐
4 Establishes the duration of the presenting illness	☐	☐	☐
5 Establishes associated history of exertional dyspnoea	☐	☐	☐
6 Establishes history of poor urine output for several days	☐	☐	☐
7 Excludes previous cardiac history and symptoms	☐	☐	☐
8 Establishes drug treatment of SLE	☐	☐	☐
9 Elicits patient's concerns and responds sensitively	☐	☐	☐
10 Uses an appropriate questioning technique	☐	☐	☐
11 Avoids or explains jargon	☐	☐	☐
12 Summarises history back to patient, including concerns	☐	☐	☐

Answers

13 Makes a reasonable attempt at a diagnosis	☐	☐	☐
14 Systematic, organised approach	☐	☐	☐

Diagnosis

Nephrotic syndrome secondary to SLE.

STATION 4.6

Patient history

I have been having increasing difficulty holding my water for the past year and wet myself more and more often. I leak when I am up and about walking or gardening and sometimes when I cough or sneeze. I don't drink and I wear a pad before going out to avoid embarrassing situations. I have no children and live alone and have been healthy all my life, except for attacks of cystitis when I was young. I am not on any drugs except for oestrogen patches to prevent hot flushes and to keep my bones healthy. This is very distressing for me and my social life is becoming increasingly restricted.

Assessment	Good	Adequate	Poor/not done
1 Appropriate introduction (full name and role)	☐	☐	☐
2 Establishes reason for patient's visit	☐	☐	☐
3 Establishes duration and associated features	☐	☐	☐
4 Establishes current medication	☐	☐	☐
5 Establishes urinary tract/pelvic infections	☐	☐	☐
6 Establishes/excludes history of abdominal surgery and/or obstetric injuries	☐	☐	☐
7 Elicits patient's concerns and responds sensitively	☐	☐	☐
8 Uses an appropriate questioning technique	☐	☐	☐
9 Avoids or explains jargon	☐	☐	☐
10 Summarises history back to the patient, including concerns	☐	☐	☐
11 Systematic, organised approach	☐	☐	☐
12 Makes a reasonable attempt at a diagnosis	☐	☐	☐

Diagnosis
Stress incontinence.

Comment

Stress incontinence in the female is caused by pelvic floor flaccidity and is usually associated with multiple pregnancies or previous obstetric trauma. Treatment is with pelvic floor exercises, to improve muscle tone. Surgical reconstruction of the pelvic floor, or implantation of a muscle stimulator, may be tried if exercises fail to work.

STATION 4.7

A

1	Testicular torsion	fig 4.7e
2	Varicocele	fig 4.7d
3	Haematocoele	fig 4.7b
4	Testicular tumour	fig 4.7c
5	Vaginal hydrocele	fig 4.7a

B

Clinical condition (diagnosis)	History	Symptoms	Signs	Treatment
1 Testicular torsion	3a	3b	1c	5d
2 Varicocele	4a	5b	4c	3d
3 Haematocele	1a	4b	2c	1d
4 Testicular tumour	2a	2b	5c	2d
5 Vaginal hydrocele	5a	1b	3c	4d

Comments

Testicular torsion is most common in childhood and is accompanied by nausea, vomiting and fever. The pain radiates to the lower abdomen.

A varicocele is caused by engorgement of the testicular venous plexus and is associated with subfertility. A haematocoele is bleeding into the testicular substance and the tunica vaginalis, usually due to blunt trauma. Evacuation of the haematoma may be necessary.

Testicular tumours produce painless enlargement: early diagnosis is essential to enable curative treatment to be initiated.

A vaginal hydrocele is a collection of fluid between the coverings of the testis and may occasionally be secondary to a testicular tumour.

STATION 4.8

Assessment	Good	Adequate	Poor/not done
1 Appropriate introduction (full name and role)	☐	☐	☐
2 Explains examination and obtains verbal consent	☐	☐	☐
3 Candidate washes their hands using the alcohol handwash provided (no marks if candidate only expresses the need to wash if handwash is provided)	☐	☐	☐
4 Ensures patient is correctly exposed and comfortable	☐	☐	☐
5 Observes patient from end of the bed – comments on presence/absence of			
Anaemia		☐	☐
Pigmentation (uraemic)		☐	☐
Dialysis catheter – CAPD/A-V fistula		☐	☐
Signs of underlying causes – diabetes, hypertension		☐	☐
6 Returns to patient's right-hand side – re-examines and comments on presence/absence of A-V fistula, peripheral stigmata of anaemia, pruritis marks, asterixis	☐	☐	☐
7 Assesses patient's face – comments on presence/absence of anaemia, facial oedema, pigmentation	☐	☐	☐
8 Assesses patient's neck for raised JVP	☐	☐	☐
9 Comments on presence/absence of scars from old 'neck lines' – jugular or subclavian	☐	☐	☐

Answers

10 Comments on presence/absence of
abdominal scars:

Nephrectomy, laparotomy ☐ ☐ ☐

CAPD catheter sites ☐ ☐ ☐

11 Correctly examines for hepatomegaly ☐ ☐ ☐

12 Correctly examines for splenomegaly ☐ ☐ ☐

13 Correctly examines the kidneys using
appropriate technique to ballot each
kidney ☐ ☐ ☐

14 Specifically checks and comments on
presence/absence of a pelvic transplanted
kidney ☐ ☐ ☐

15 Assesses for ascites – using correct/
appropriate technique ☐ ☐ ☐

16 Specifically assesses for and comments
on the presence/absence of aortic, renal
and femoral bruits ☐ ☐ ☐

17 Completes examination by checking for
peripheral oedema and peripheral pulses ☐ ☐ ☐

18 Covers patient and leaves them
comfortable, thanks patient ☐ ☐ ☐

19 Asks examiner for results of BP, BM and
urinalysis ☐ ☐ ☐

20 Presents findings in a fluent, logical
manner ☐ ☐ ☐

Answers

Examiner asks

'What are the common causes of chronic renal failure in a patient of this age?'

- Young adults: diabetes; APCKD, toxins, sepsis
- Middle age: diabetes, toxins, infection, malignancy
- Older adults: diabetes; hypertension; malignancy
- All: causes of nephritic/nephrotic syndrome

What three blood investigation results would you like to know and why?

- FBC: Hb – anaemia; WCC – infection or malignancy
- U&ES: K^+ high to hyperkalaemia; urea and creatinine
- Corrected calcium: low, phosphate- high
- Albumin: low
- HCO_3^- assess for acidosis

What are the indications for emergency dialysis in a known dialysis patient?

- K^+> 6.5 mmol/l
- Signs of fluid overload
- Worsening acidosis
- Pericardial rub

Answers

STATION 4.9

1 **True** – the raised haemoglobin and haematocrit are consistent with polycythaemia.

2 **True** – adult polycystic kidney disease and renal carcinoma may both produce excessive erythropoetin causing polycythaemia.

3 **False** – this is suggestive of lower urinary tract infection and may be associated with symptoms of cystitis.

4 **False** – these results are consistent with a normochromic, normocytic anaemia.

5 **True** – chronic renal disorders are commonly associated with an anaemia of chronic disease.

6 **False** – anaemia of chronic disease is associated with a normal plasma ferretin.

7 **True** – in this case malignancy of the renal tract must be excluded.

8 **False** – these results are suggestive of an ongoing bleeding disorder. This would be in keeping with a renal tract problem causing chronic haematuria eg polycystic kidney disease or renal carcinoma. Renal abscesses do not usually present in this manner.

9 **True** – the raised platelet count in association with the microcytic anaemia is consistent with an active bleeding problem.

10 **True** – this patient has results consistent with multiple myeloma. The four investigations of choice are plasma calcium (raised), plasma electrophoresis (monoclonal bands), ESR > 100, urinary Bence–Jones proteins.

11 **False** – myeloma is associated with hypercalcaemia.

12 **False** – the plasma cells noted are seen in the peripheral blood film of 15% of patients with myeloma.

Answers

STATION 4.10

1 **False** – the results are suggestive of pre-renal impairment. The urea is raised disproportionately higher than the creatinine.

2 **True** – a GI bleed will cause hypovolaemia, leading to pre-renal impairment. It will also cause a rise in the urea due to the absorption of protein from blood in the gut.

3 **False** – the low urea is not compatible with dehydration.

4 **False** – this blood result is consistent with blood drawn from a vein proximal to a dextrose infusion. There are no suggestions of renal impairment despite the hyperglycaemia.

5 **True** – the patient has diabetic nephropathy. The raised HBA1c suggests poorly controlled diabetes. The low bicarbonate shows a metabolic acidosis which would be consistent with chronic renal disease.

6 **True** – this is the classical lesion of diabetic glomerulosclerosis.

7 **True** – initial treatment of the hyperkalaemia should be with insulin and dextrose. However this is a short-term solution and in view of the patient's renal failure the best treatment would be dialysis.

8 **False** – the patient has acute on chronic renal failure with a low serum calcium. These data do not support a diagnosis of myeloma. Renal failure in myeloma may result from a nephrotic syndrome, obstruction of the nephrons due to heavy light chain excretion, amyloidosis, melamatous infiltration of the kidneys and the associated hypercalcaemia and hyperuricaemia.

9 **False** – this patient has obstructive nephropathy secondary to prostatic carcinoma.

10 **True** – this is an important investigation in a patient with prostatic carcinoma which commonly metastasises to bone.

Answers

STATION 4.11

1 (B)

This urine culture has grown acid fast bacilli, proving this woman has renal tract tuberculosis. This requires at least six months of antituberculosis treatment.

2 (E)

Although there is significant growth of pseudomonas, the white cell count indicates this is most likely to be a contaminant. Unless the patient is unwell this should not be treated with antibiotics.

3 (D)

This patient has renal colic secondary to recurrent stones. The specimen shows a sterile pyuria. Other causes include interstitial nephritis, papillary necrosis and tuberculosis of the renal tract.

4 (C)

This microscopy shows renal red cell casts which are indicative of renal disease. The history is suggestive of renal failure with a possible nephrotic syndrome.

5 (A)

E. coli is a common organism causing urinary tract infections. Other common causes of UTI include *Proteus*, *Staphylococcus saprophyticus* or *epidermis* and *Klebsiella.*

STATION 4.12

(1) **(E) (b)**

The malar rash is characteristic of SLE as are the anti-ds DNA antibodies. Several other auto-antibodies are found in SLE which have now been linked to specific subsets within the disease, eg anticardiolipin antibody, anti-ro and anti-la. SLE is commonly associated with renal involvement and may present with asymptomatic proteinuria or an acute glomerulonephritis with nephritic or nephrotic syndrome.

(2) **(D) (a)**

The significance of the hepatitis B antigen in PAN is still unclear. It occurs in a small percentage of patients with the disorder and is thought to indicate a possible environmental association with the vasculitis.

(3) **(A) (e)**

Systemic sclerosis (scleroderma) has now been reclassified into two separate sub-groups.

Limited cutaneous sceleroderma, previously called the CREST syndrome, is most readily identified by the anticentromere antibody, whereas **diffuse cutaneous sceleroderma** is associated with the anti-Scl 70 antibody. Patients with diffuse disease commonly develop renal involvement principally manifested as severe hypertension and worsening cardiac failure.

(4) **(B) (c)**

The patient has signs of both renal and lower respiratory tract involvement consistent with glomerular basement membrane disease or Goodpasture's disease. With the advent of immunofluorescence microscopy it became evident that the original syndrome described by Goodpasture in the USA after the influenza epidemic in 1918 was in fact common to several disorders including the systemic vasculitides. The antibody shares a common antigen in the glomerular basement membrane and the alveolar basement membrane. This has now been localised to type IV collagen which is a major component of both membranes.

(5) **(C) (d)**

Antineutrophil cytoplasmic antibodies (ANCA) are subdivided into cANCA (c = cytoplasmic) and pANCA (p = perinuclear) according to their pattern of indirect immunofluorescence. cANCA is closely linked to Wegener's granulonmatosis and more recently has been specifically linked to the antigen proteinase 3. The presence of antiproteinase 3 antibodies is now regarded as diagnostic of Wegener's granulomatosis. pANCA is associated with microscopic PAN and has been linked to the antigen myeloperoxidase. This is not as specific as the association of cANCA and proteinase 3; it is seen in several other disorders, including inflammatory bowel disease and autoimmune hepatitis.

Answers

STATION 4.13

(1) (a) **True**   (b) **False**   (c) **True**   (d) **True**   (e) **False**

This is a plain abdominal radiograph of the abdomen showing grossly enlarged renal outlines (fig 4.13a). The normal kidneys should be no more than three lumbar vertebrae in length. Causes of bilaterally enlarged kidneys include polycystic kidney disease, bilateral malignant tumours and hydronephrosis. The lower pole of the right kidney has a clear area of calcification which should be considered malignant until proven otherwise. This patient has polycystic kidney disease and this appearance may be caused by calcification of haemorrhage into one of the cysts. However, renal ultrasound, IVP and urinary cytology should be performed.

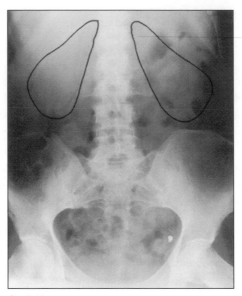

fig 4.13a

(2) (a) **False**   (b) **False**   (c) **False**   (d) **True**   (e) **True**

This plain abdominal radiograph shows a large staghorn calculus in the pelvis of the right kidney. Such calculi are associated with recurrent UTIs particularly with *Proteus* infections. These organisms hydrolyse urea and so cause alkylisation of the urine which in turn favours stone formation. The majority of renal stones are composed of calcium oxalate and phosphate, the others being composed of uric acid, cystine and magnesium ammonium phosphate.

(3) (a) **True**   (b) **False**   (c) **False**   (d) **True**   (e) **True**

This view from an IVP shows a huge vesical calculus within the bladder. The two ureters are dilated (hydroureters) due to the bladder obstruction being caused by the stone. The right pelvicalyceal system in particular shows evidence of 'clubbing' also resulting from the obstruction. Bladder stones formation is related to foreign bodies, eg indwelling catheters, within the bladder and bladder outflow tract obstruction. The majority of patients have stagnation of urine within the bladder and significant bacteruria.

STATION 4.14

1 Right-sided Staghorn renal calculus.
2 Obstruction to drainage of the renal pelvis and progressive destruction of the renal parenchyma from pressure and infection.
3 Fragmentation with shockwave lithotripsy and surgical removal of the calculus, together with treatment of any underlying infection. Nephrectomy may be required if the kidney is irretrievably damaged.

Comment

Staghorn calculi are shaped by, and virtually fill, the entire pelvicalyceal system. Symptoms such as back pain and renal colic occur when the calculi obstruct one or more calyces or the renal pelvis.

Most renal calculi are visible on plain radiography; only pure uric acid stones and the rare xanthine and 'protein matrix' stones are radiolucent.

Answers

STATION 4.15

1 Radio-opaque vesical (bladder) calculi
2 Dietary factors
    Metabolic (hereditary) cause
    Chronic cystitis
3 Transurethral removal of the calculus after crushing with a lithotrite or fragmentation with shock-wave lithotripsy

Comment

Calcium-containing urinary stones are far more frequently encountered in Western society than areuric acid or phosphate stones. Metabolic evaluation is undertaken if active stone disease is suspected, ie evidence of new stone formation, stone growth or passage of gravel within one year. Absorptive hypercalcaemia is associated with an altered bowel response to vitamin D, leading to increased absorption of calcium, elevated serum calcium levels and depression of parathyroid function, with increased urinary excretion of calcium. Renal hypercalcaemia is due to the inability of the kidney to conserve calcium, due to a tubular functional defect. This leads to a low serum calcium level, resulting in stimulation of parathyroid hormone secretion and increased synthesis of vitamin D, with increased absorption of calcium from the bowel and resorption from bone.

STATION 4.16

1 Intravenous urogram (IVU)
2 Bilateral duplex kidneys and ureters
3 Retrograde uretero-pyelogram
4 A urinary tract infection destroying pelvicalyceal system; other possibilities include ureteric calculus originating in the abnormal pelvicalyceal system

Comment

Pelvi-ureteric congenital abnormalities are not uncommon and range from complete absence to duplication or triplication of the renal pelvis and ureter. They may cause obstruction requiring urgent treatment, or they may be asymptomatic and of no clinical significance. Obstruction at the pelvi-ureteric junction is due to a developmental abnormality that requires surgical correction. Obstruction at the uretero-vescal junction is four times more common in boys than in girls. Surgery is usually indicated, with excision of the distal ureter and uretal reimplantaion.

STATION 4.17

1 Intravenous urography (pyelography)
2 Hydrocalices and hydropelvis of right kidney
   Obstruction at the pelvi-ureteric junction
3 Surgical reconstruction of the pelvi-ureteric junction
4 Pressure necrosis of the renal cortex, with or without pyelonephritis

Comment

On presentation this patient would have had a KUB (plain radiograph) followed by an ultrasound scan of the right collecting system. The latter is usually diagnostic in obstructive uropathies. An IVU demonstrates the anatomical details of the site of obstruction for surgical reconstruction.

STATION 4.18

1 (a) This is a renal angiogram showing a downwardly displaced left kidney with a highly vascularised area above it. These appearances may be due to a malignant tumour or polycystic disease.

   (b) Indications for this investigation include suspected renal artery stenosis, intrarenal arterial disease, eg polyarteritis nodosa, which causes intrarenal aneurysms, and defining the presence and extent of a renal tumour.
   (c) Important questions to ask the patient prior to starting this procedure should include identifying the patient, the procedure they are to have and the reason for it, identifying previous allergies to contrast media and drug allergies.

2 (a) This is a plain abdominal radiograph of the abdomen showing calcification of the right kidney.

   (b) Common causes of renal calcification include:

   Diffuse: medullary sponge kidney, hypercalcaemia and renal tubular acidosis.
   Medullary: as diffuse and papillary necrosis
   Cortical: acute cortical necrosis, chronic transplant rejection
   Focal areas: tuberculosis, renal carcinoma, polycystic disease and amyloidosis

3 (a) This is an IVU.
   (b) It shows a right pelvic kidney without functioning normal kidneys. The bones of the pelvis show evidence of renal osteopathy.
   (c) These abnormalities indicate a renal transplant following chronic renal failure.

Answers

There are two tablets in the stomach. The bone changes associated with renal failure are termed 'renal osteodystrophy'. Renal osteodystrophy initially arises due to osteomalacia associated with chronic renal failure. Hypocalcaemia leads to secondary and subsequent tertiary hyperparathyroidism. The classical 'rugger jersey spine' of tertiary hyperparathyroidism, which is alternating hypo- and hyperdense bands within the vertebrae is not apparent in this film.

STATION 4.19

fig 4.19b: shows a downwardly displaced left sided kidney. The right kidney is not as well visualised but is within normal limits as is the bladder. This appearance may be caused by a large renal mass displacing the kidney. Examples include renal cell carcinoma, large renal cysts and polycystic renal disease.

fig 4.19c: the left renal pelvicalyceal system is grossly dilated. This appearance is consistent with pelvi-ureteric obstruction. This may be caused by a functional abnormality arising due to an inelastic ring of tissue at the junction, strictures, transitional cell carcinoma and calculi.

fig 4.19d: this is a bilateral abnormality demonstrating a horseshoe kidney. Both pelvicalyceal systems are rotated through 90 degrees, appearing to be 'end on'. This is characteristic and arises due to an embryonic failure of the developing kidneys to split apart as they ascend along their development pathways in the abdomen to their normal positions. The disorder may affect a small area, such as the lower poles or may include the kidney's entire length.

fig 4.19e: this IVU shows an irregular area at the insertion of the right ureter into the bladder with no visible ureter or kidney above it. This implies a non-functioning right kidney due to obstruction within the bladder. Further investigation revealed a transitional cell carcinoma of the bladder.

STATION 4.20

(A) Lumbar vertebra   (E) Small bowel
(B) Abdominal aorta   (F) Liver
(C) Inferior vena cava   (G) Spleen
(D) Left kidney   (H) Right renal tumour

STATION 4.21

1 Urodynamic (pressure-flow) studies
2 Detrusor instability
   Prostatic hyperplasia
   Bladder neck hypertrophy
   Neurogenic bladder
3 Voluntary micturition commences at X and ends at Y

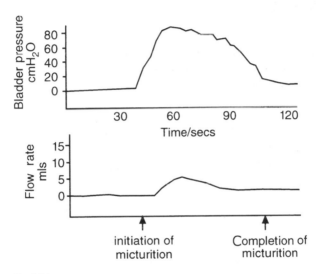

fig 4.21

Comment

The patient has a double-lumen indwelling catheter – one for filling the bladder and the other for pressure measurement. A catheter in the rectum monitors abdominal pressure changes. The latter is subtracted from the bladder pressure recording to give the true intravesical pressure.

The bladder catheter is removed prior to voiding and a flow meter attached to the commode monitors the volume of urine voided and computes the flow rate in ml/s.

STATION 4.22

1 Enalapril, bumetanide, amoxycillin , aspirin and diclofenac – penicillins and NSAIDs may cause an acute tubulo-interstitial nephritis. This patient has evidence of mild renal impairment and has known IHD which may point to an element of atherosclerotic renal artery stenosis. This should make one wary about adding in an ACE inhibitor to this patient's regime

2 Gliclazide (sulphonylurea) ; acarbose (alpha glucosidase inhibitor).

3 Amoxycillin, omeprazole, aspirin and diclofenac may all be directly contributing to her nausea

4 Enalapril, bumetanide, GTN spray – may all cause postural hypotension. Aspirin and diclofenac may lead to acute and chronic gastrointestinal blood loss, indirectly contributing to her hypotension

5 FBC – to exclude anaemia

Glucose and HBA_{1c} – diabetic control

Lipid profile – if not checked recently

Calcium and phosphate – essential in chronic renal impairment.

USS of the renal tract – principally to exclude obstruction

Urinalysis – to exclude red cell casts

MSU – to exclude urinary tract infection. This may be contributing to her worsening renal function

STATION 4.23

(1) **(D) (c)**

Benign prostatic hyperplasia (BPH), is a histological diagnosis which may be inferred from a patient's history and a normal PSA, but must be confirmed by cystoscopic biopsy of the prostate. If symptoms are mild or the patient is not fit for surgical intervention a 5α reductase inhibitor, such as finasteride may be used. 5α Reductase is an enzyme required for the production of testosterone, which is known to worsen BPH.

(2) **(F) (e)**

Patients with chronic renal failure commonly suffer with a normochromic/normocytic anaemia. This anaemia is frequently due to loss of erythropoetin production in the failing kidneys. Although this is a common disorder among this group of patients, not all respond to erythropoetin replacement. All such patients should have haemetinics, ie vitamin B_{12}, folate and ferritin to exclude other, more readily treatable causes. It should be noted that erythropoietin treatment was one of the first drugs to be withheld on financial reasoning alone.

(3) **(B) (e)**

Prostatic carcinoma is a common malignancy of older men, although it can occur from age 40. The diagnosis is inferred on history, examination, which may show a 'craggy', abnormal prostate, and investigation may show deranged U+Es and raised PSA. Metastatic disease may be apparent on CXR, USS of the liver and on bone scan. Diagnosis is confirmed on prostatic biopsy.

Treatment is principally surgical resection with or without bilateral orchidectomy. Anti-androgens such as cyproterone, are commonly used in inoperable cases, as are other treatments to lower circulating testosterone, eg stilboestrol and LHRH injections.

(4) **(C) (f)**

Urinary incontinence may have many causes, one of which is detrusor instability, leading to poor bladder sphincter control. This disorder is readily treated with anticholinergics such as oxybutinin. However, the treatment should not be instituted until a postmicturition residual bladder volume has been measured. If this is greater than 150 to 200 ml, the addition of an anticholinergic will worsen the condition as it will cause urinary retention, stagnation and infection.

(5) **(A) (d)**

Diabetic patients, particularly those with hypertension, should be treated with an ACE inhibitor. The newer generation of ACE inhibitors, eg quinapril, lisinopril and perindopril, retard and possibly reverse both microvascular changes and atherosclerotic disease.

(6) **(E) (b)**

Patients with myelo- and lymphoproliferative disorders are particularly at risk of gout due to the massive turnover of cells in these conditions. Allopurinol is often given prophylactically to these patients to stop overt clinical gout arising. It should be remembered that hyperuricaemia is 20–30 times more common than clinical gout.

Answers

STATION 4.24

Assessment	Good	Adequate	Poor/not done
1 Cleaning and draping of the region	☐	☐	☐
2 Catheterisation technique (non-touch; use of lubricant)	☐	☐	☐
3 Ensures the catheter tip is in the bladder by drawing out the urine before blowing up the balloon	☐	☐	☐
4 Checks balloon volume size; blows up catheter balloon with the appropriate amount of saline	☐	☐	☐
5 Connects catheter to drainage bag	☐	☐	☐

Comment

When catheterising to relieve acute or acute on chronic urinary retention, choosing the smallest gauge self-retaining catheter (CH 9, 10 or 12) minimises urethral mucosal trauma. Check the balloon volume size before commencing. When blowing up the balloon in a Foley catheter ensure that the catheter tip is well in the bladder to avoid blowing up the balloon in the urethra.

STATION 4.25

1 A: Puncture needle
   B: Catheter with sleeve
   C: Adaptor – clamp
2 Percutaneous suprapubic catheterization
3 Urinary retention (usually acute)
   (a) A distended, readily palpable urinary bladder

Comment

This is a bedside surgical procedure undertaken under local anaesthesia, to relieve acute or chronic retension, often following failed transurethral catheterisation. A fully sterile technique must be adopted and the procedure must not be undertaken if the bladder is not palpable.

Answers

STATION 4.26

Patient histories

Husband: I am a 35-year-old sales rep for a pharmaceutical firm. We have been married for four years and have two children. We do not wish to add to our family, and my wife and I have discussed the various methods of birth control between ourselves and with our GP, and vasectomy is the procedure we have agreed on. I am healthy and fit and am not on medication. Ten years ago I was treated for TB of the lung and made a full recovery; a right-sided groin hernia was repaired four years ago.

Wife: I am 28 years old and am a housewife. Our children are one and three years of age. I have a seven-year-old daughter from a previous marriage, and she lives with her father and stepmother. My husband and I have completed our family and do not want any more children. I tried the birth control pill many years ago and suffered side-effects. I used a birth control coil after my last child but had to have it removed six months ago, as it caused heavy and painful periods. My husband and I have talked about the vasectomy operation for some time now, and our GP agrees that this operation would be the best for us.

Assessment	Good	Adequate	Poor/not done
1 Appropriate introduction (full name and role)	☐	☐	☐
2 Explains purpose of the interview	☐	☐	☐
3 Checks with both partners the reason for attending the clinic	☐	☐	☐
4 Ascertains reason for request:			
Completed family	☐	☐	☐
Other methods ineffective	☐	☐	☐
5 Ascertains other methods of contraception tried:			
Side-effects: groin haematoma, sperm granuloma	☐	☐	☐
Failures: sterility is not immediate recanalisation rare	☐	☐	☐

6 Establishes understanding of irrevocable
   nature of the procedure ☐ ☐ ☐

7 Reconfirms that both partners understand
   the procedure ☐ ☐ ☐

8 Takes care to include both partners in
   the interview ☐ ☐ ☐

9 Uses an appropriate questioning technique ☐ ☐ ☐

10 Avoids or explains jargon ☐ ☐ ☐

11 Systematic, organised approach ☐ ☐ ☐

Comment

When filling in a consent form for vasectomy both (married) partners must be in agreement in wishing to have the procedure carried out. They must also understand the irreversible nature of the operation. Sterility is not assured until three consecutive semen samples taken over three months after the vasectomy are azoospermic. This fact must be emphasised during consent, and an alternative form of contraception should be used in the interim period.

Answers

Mock Exam

The table contains six examinations of 19 stations taken from the text, each lasts two hours – this allows three five minute rest stations in examinations 2–4, and two in examination 5. The symbol + indicates a 10, rather than the usual 5, minute station, and ++ an extra 5 minute preparation for a 10 minute station. A 'subject' is needed to give the history, where this is provided in the text answer, and also for examination stations when stated.

Station	1	2	3	4	5	6
1	1.1	1.5	1.3	1.2+	1.4	1.7
2	1.6+	1.10	1.9	1.8+	1.14+	1.11+
3	1.15+	1.18	1.13+	1.12+	1.16+	1.20
4	1.19	1.23	1.17	1.22	1.21	1.24
5	1.26	1.27	1.28	1.31	1.25	1.30
6	2.1	1.36+	1.34	2.6	1.32	1.33
7	2.7+	2.8+	2.3	2.13+	2.4	2.5
8	2.9	2.10	2.11	2.16	2.12	2.14
9	2.19	2.20	2.18+	2.23	2.17+	2.15+
10	2.25	2.26	2.21	2.29	2.22	2.24
11	2.31+	2.32+	2.27	2.35	2.30	2.28++
12	2.38	2.39	2.33+	2.41	2.34+	2.36
13	3.1	3.3	2.40	3.6	2.42	3.9
14	3.14	3.15	3.2	3.7	3.4	3.10
15	3.17	3.18	3.8	3.12	3.13	3.16
16	4.1	4.2	3.11	4.5	4.3	4.6
17	4.7	4.8+	4.4+	4.11	4.10	4.12
18	4.13	4.14	4.9	4.17	4.16	4.18
19	4.21	4.24	4.15	4.25	4.23	4.26

The OSCE marking scheme

Traditionally, academic assessment has been 'norm' referenced, whereby candidates are compared to one another and are ranked from the best to the worst. In recent years the value of 'norm' referencing has come under question and 'criterion' referencing has become more accepted.

Criterion-referenced assessment is not new, the most obvious examples being the driving test and swimming life saving assessments. In both these examples a candidate must demonstrate a 'minimum competency level' for the given skills, ie driving a motor vehicle or saving a drowning person. Unlike traditional, norm-referenced assessment, there is no division of candidates into excellent, good, average, unsatisfactory and poor; there is only pass (competent) and fail (not competent).

Criterion referencing is easily applied to the OSCE format. A committee of examiners meets several months prior to the examinations and, through discussion, sets a minimum competency score, ie a passing score, for each given station. This score reflects what a candidate taking the OSCE should be reasonably expected to achieve, given their expected core knowledge, the time restrictions and the stress of the examination. These, in turn, should be reflected in the validity of the OSCE.

In volumes 1 and 2 the checklists are divided into three columns headed **Good**, **Adequate** and **Poor/not done**. These headings subdivide students into good, average and poor, where poor candidates do not demonstrate an acceptable level of competence, i.e. fail. However, in many medical establishments, the division of good and average candidates is regarded as old fashioned, regressing back to norm referencing and therefore the headings may read **Adequate or competent**, **Attempted but unsatisfactory** and **Not done**.

Some medical colleges apply weighting of individual items within a checklist. For instance, the initial item on each checklist 'Appropriate introduction (full name and role)', may have a maximum score of two marks if performed well, whereas another item, eg auscultating the four areas of the heart correctly, may carry 5 marks if performed well. Both would be given a lesser mark if performed adequately and 0 marks if not done at all. We have chosen not to weight individual items in our checklists. This is because:

(i)   We feel that weighting of items in this way does not improve the discriminatory power of the examination.

(ii)   We think students should be discerning enough to realise which are the important key points that will be more heavily weighted in a checklist.

We have, therefore, generally used 3 columns for our checklists, **Good, Adequate** and **Poor/not done**, carrying 3, 2 and 0 marks respectively. Certain checklists, however, only have 2 columns, i.e. Adequate and Not done. These are typically items which are required to be named, e.g. risk factors for a DVT or contraindications to a given treatment. One can only mention them or not and for this reason a 'good' column' is not applicable. In such cases 1 mark is given for adequate column and zero for the Poor/not done column.

To obtain the total score

For each station, minimum competency or pass mark is calculated by a committee of examiners/experts. If a candidate scores each item as 'adequate' this will equate to the 'pass' mark. A candidate should therefore aim to get an adequate or good for each item. If one scores adequate or poor/not done in the majority of items, this implies a lack of knowledge or areas of weakness and should be used to direct the student's learning.

In most OSCEs the stations are deemed to be as important as one another, so that the mean pass mark of the total number of stations is taken as the pass mark for the overall examination. If individual stations are important in terms of 'must pass', a weighting system may be applied to calculate the overall pass mark.

We have used one other style of marking whereby the station poses a series of questions to the student regarding an investigation, e.g. an abdominal radiograph, or a given scenario, e.g. management of a head injury patient. Examiners may consider that such answers should also carry serious consequences for the candidate, such as an outright failure on that question.

Establishing rapport with a patient is essential in a doctor-patient relationship. At the initial meeting, greetings and introductions help to put the patient at ease and ensure patient co-operation with the history and/or examination. In these stations, therefore, marks are allocated for such interaction. Positive criteria include empathy, putting a patient at their ease and establishing their confidence by careful listening and responding to verbal and non-verbal cues.

Revision Checklist

Gastroenterology

Tongue – leukplakia and cancer ☐
Parotid gland tumours ☐
Oesophageal carcinoma ☐
Gastro-oesophageal reflux disease (GORD) ☐
Peptic ulcer disease ☐
Gastric cancer ☐
The acute abdomen ☐
Viral hepatitis ☐
Portal hypertension and cirrhosis ☐
Cholecystitis ☐
Pancreatitis ☐
Inflammatory bowel disease ☐
Diverticular disease ☐
Colonic polyps and cancer ☐
Piles, fissures and fistulae ☐

Neurology and Psychiatry

Headache ☐
Meningititis and encephalitis ☐
Seizures ☐
Meningomyelocoele and hydrocephalus ☐
Hypothalmic and pituitary lesions ☐
Stroke disease ☐
Multiple sclerosis ☐
Parkinson's disease ☐
Cranial nerve disease ☐
Motor neurone disease ☐
Peripheral neuropathy and nerve injuries ☐
Alcohol and drug abuse ☐
Eating disorders ☐
Depression ☐
Personality disorders ☐
Mania ☐
Schizophrenia ☐

Ophthalmology and Otolaryngology

Eye injuries ☐

The red eye ☐

Uveitis ☐

Glaucoma ☐

Cataract ☐

Retinopathy ☐

Otitis media ☐

Glue ear ☐

Chronic sinusitis ☐

Epistaxis ☐

Tonsilitis/ pharyngitis ☐

Urology and Renal Medicine

Urinary tract infections ☐

Haematuria ☐

Prostate hypertrophy and carcinoma ☐

Urinary incontinence ☐

Urinary retention ☐

Renal calculus disease ☐

Renal failure ☐

Diabetic nephrology ☐

Glomerulo nephritis and nephrotic syndrome ☐

Polycystic kidney disease ☐

Recommended Reading List

Medical Texts

Hutchinson's Clinical Methods: Hutchinson R and Swash M, 21st edition, W B Saunders 2001.

Davidson's Principles and Practice of Medicine: Edwards CRW, Bouchier IAD, Haslett C and Chilvers ER (editors), 19th edition, Churchill Livingstone 2002.

Clinical Medicine: Kumar P and Clark M (editors), 5th edition, Saunders 2002.

Lecture Notes on Dermatology: Graham-Brown RAC, Burns T, 8th edition, Blackwell Science 2002.

Examining Patients: An Introduction to Clinical Medicine: Toghill PJ (editor), 2nd edition, Edward Arnold 1994.

Lecture Notes on Clinical Medicine: Rubenstein D, Bradley JR and Wayne D, 6th edition, Blackwell Science 2002.

Surgical Texts

Hamilton Bailey's Demonstrations of Physical Signs in Clinical Surgery: Lumley JSP, 18th edition, Butterworth Heinemann 1997.

Lecture Notes on General Surgery: Watson JE, Ellis H and Calne R, 10th edition, Blackwell Science 2002.

The Washington Manual of Surgery: Doherty GM (editor), 2nd edition, Lippincott, Williams and Wilkins 1999.

Bailey and Love's Short Practice of Surgery: Russell RCG, Williams NS, Bulstrode CJK (editors), 24th edition, Hodder Arnold 2004.

Obstetrics and Gynaecology Texts

ABC of Antenatal Care: Chamberlain G, Morgan M, 4th edition, BMJ 2002.

Lecture Notes in Obstetrics and Gynaecology: Hamilton-Fairley, D, 2nd edition, Blackwell Science 2004.

Index